POLYVAGAL
THEORY
MADE
SIMPLE

70 SELF GUIDED EXERCISES

TO QUICKLY STIMULATE YOUR VAGUS NERVE, EASE ANXIETY

FOR NERVOUS SYSTEM REGULATION & HELP RELEASE TRAUMA

CALVIN CAUFIELD

Table of Contents

"Earth will be safe when we feel in us enough safety."

(Thich Nhat Hanh)

Your Journey Into Safety

What if I told you that there is a nerve in your body that when stimulated could help make you feel safe? That there are physiological tools and practices you can do on your own that can help you feel more grounded, more connected, reduce stress, and, over time, even help release trauma? Wouldn't you like to know more?

I definitely did when I first heard about the Polyvagal Theory (PVT) in 2018. At that time, many practitioners around me started speaking about this theory developed by Stephen Porges, PhD, in 1994.[1] Many were already successfully applying its principles and techniques in sessions with clients. I saw cases of chronic pain patients finally getting better after years of unsuccessful treatments with classic therapy and medication; even traumatized patients were able to slowly work through and release deep, unprocessed memories and emotions. It seemed like one big mystery, and as someone who had been supporting clients for many years myself, I was intrigued. Three decades after Porges introduced this revolutionary approach of integrating the body into the healing of trauma and stress-related illnesses, science is yet to catch up with explaining how PVT works exactly. Those actually working with PVT—licensed psychotherapists, psychologists, counselors, body workers and alternative healers—all seem to have no doubt about its effectiveness.

This workbook is intended to unravel some of the principles around PVT, and how physiological interventions of the longest nerve in the body can help bring about states of deeper relaxation, calm, even healing and release. According to Porges, we can trigger our bodies to feel safe and, over time, reduce stress responses, even releasing trauma.[2] We now have the understanding that many more people are affected by one-time, multiple-time, or long-lasting trauma than we previously thought. Trauma and its immediate and long-term consequences are everywhere, and those affected have no choice but to eventually embark on their personal healing paths if they are longing to overcome traumatic experiences and the negative consequences on body, emotions and mind.

Who is This Workbook For?

This workbook is for everyone who is curious to find out more, discover and experience alternative approaches to healing, or who is already convinced of the effectiveness of PVT as a patient or a professional. All the tools and practices that are introduced in this workbook can really be tried out by anyone. At times, it may become supportive or even necessary to seek external support, especially if you are exploring this workbook for your own deeper healing by overcoming trauma. Quite often people are able to successfully deal with difficult situations better than they expect or assume, but should you ever find yourself overwhelmed or not capable of dealing with thoughts, emotions or sensations that are arising, please seek external support.

This workbook cannot replace professional psychotherapy. You are invited to move through this book at your own pace, choosing to try the tools that you are most excited about and feel ready for. Gift yourself a separate journal, one that is appealing to you, as you make your way through this workbook. Journaling is one of the easiest, cheapest and most effective ways to support your personal healing process.[3]

What content can you expect? In the first part of this workbook, you can expect a brief yet solid introduction to the principles and functioning of PVT. You will find out about your nervous system, the vagus nerve and the three different states according to PVT. We will also explore the characteristics of a regulated vs. dysregulated nervous system, and briefly visit the different conditions PVT is currently used for. In *Parts 3* and *4*, you will be introduced to an array of powerful and effective practices around using PVT to self-regulate and even work with trauma. Tools will mainly focus on working with breath and touch. In *Part 4*, our focus is on tools and practices to support co-regulation, and to enable us to be the happy and healthy social beings that we are intended to be.

Throughout the workbook, you will find references to scientific findings and experts where they exist, and you will continue learning about PVT and the nervous system as we move forward. Some of the tools can also be found as audio recordings. You will find a specific text note in these cases. Get ready to learn things about your body and physiology that you didn't know and that you are much more in control of your feelings, emotions and stress responses than you think! An exciting journey lies ahead for you. All that is needed from you is a certain openness and curiosity to new ideas and concepts, the availability to try things out, and the discernment to differentiate between topics that can be solved on your own versus those that need further support and attention. Embarking on a healing journey is a brave step into living a life of more joy, aliveness and connection. Everyone is worthy of such a life. I truly hope you enjoy this workbook!

PART 1

Polyvagal Theory in Simple Words

L et's dive right into this first part by helping you gain a solid and clear understanding of the Polyvagal Theory (PVT). Looking at the word "polyvagal," *poly* means many, and *vagal* is referring to the vagus nerve, originating from the Latin word for wander. The vagus nerve is a cranial nerve, coming directly from the brain, and is a core component of the autonomic nervous system (ANS), specifically the parasympathetic nervous system. Your ANS operates your internal organs, and is constantly receiving and interpreting information from your body and the external environment to identify whether you are safe or if there is a threat. The ANS is split into the sympathetic and parasympathetic nervous system, the first being responsible for the so-called fight and flight response, and the latter for what is known as the rest and digest response.

All of these mechanisms are designed to keep us safe and help us survive, so if there is an external event or trigger that is potentially threatening, the nervous system helps us react. The traditional understanding of such a reaction to a threat, our stress reaction, was to compare it to a light switch: The body was either stressed or not stressed. Porges noticed that some of his patients seemed to be in a parasympathetic reaction (not stressed), yet they were not happy or did not seem really relaxed. From there, he suggested three different responses of the autonomic nervous system that we assume according to our perceived safety. Take note that only the first response is a response of safety.

1. **Parasympathetic ventral vagal:** relaxed, safe response
2. **Sympathetic:** mobilized fight or flight response
3. **Parasympathetic dorsal vagal:** immobilized frozen or collapsed response

Let's look at each of these three responses in more detail. **1. Parasympathetic ventral vagal** is our happy place. Here we feel relaxed, calm and are open for social engagement with others. **2. Sympathetic activation** is actually what most people associate with stress. It can be characterized by feelings of worry, anxiety and agitation, and we either try to fight whatever is stressing us, or we try to run away. In this more hyperactive state, we can also build up a lot of tension in our muscles without even knowing it (a potential explanation for chronic pain where no cause can be found). **3. Parasympathetic dorsal vagal** is characterized by immobilization that can either look like a total collapse or freeze response. We are likely to feel stuck, lethargic or hopeless, lacking motivation and drive. From a physical perspective, the body may also be more flaccid, hanging softly and loosely. This response is also called dorsal vagal shutdown. Porges suggested these responses do not happen consciously, and people may assume hybrid reactions, consisting of mobility and immobility, for example.

Deb Dana, a colleague of Porges, uses the analogy of a ladder to explain the relationship and hierarchy between the different responses. Imagine the following scenario: You are walking in nature and are in your happy place in a ventral vagal activation. All of a sudden you hear something moving in the bushes. Then you see a pretty large snake moving onto the pathway and stopping just in front of you. Automatically, you move into sympathetic activation as cortisol is being released, your pulse and heartbeat go up and blood gets pumped into the limbs as you are ready to react. After a short stop, the snake continues and leaves the path, disappearing into the bushes on the other side. You take a few more moments, then you relax back into ventral vagal response and continue your walk. In the graphic below, you can see the hierarchy and the simplified wording of ventral vagal, sympathetic and dorsal vagal I will use moving forward.

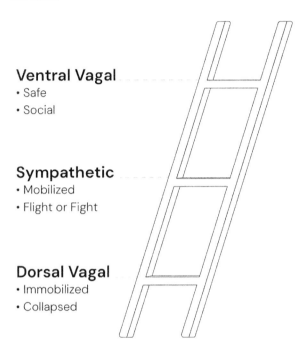

Ventral Vagal
• Safe
• Social

Sympathetic
• Mobilized
• Flight or Fight

Dorsal Vagal
• Immobilized
• Collapsed

In this specific situation, it's easy to come back up the ladder right away because the snake left immediately. Now, what happens with prolonged stress or traumatic situations in our lives where the stressor or trigger is there for a prolonged period of time? When we are in sympathetic activation, so much adrenaline and cortisol are released that this cannot be sustained for a long time. At some point, the sympathetic nervous system is maxed out, and our will to survive will cause another response, moving us further down the ladder and leading to the dorsal vagal response or shutdown, in which we freeze and eventually collapse. It's important to understand that for healing and trauma processing, we need to eventually come up the ladder again. For most people, this also includes moving through sympathetic responses on their way back to safety during ventral vagal activation. It is important to note that from an evolutionary perspective, these different responses mentioned above have developed millions of years apart, with social responses and engagement being much later responses than the shut-down response.

Today, many of our lives are characterized by constant, even chronic, stress (noise, traffic, electronics, constant influx of information and constant availability, work, parenting, etc.). Life has become a lot more stressful than it was back in the savanna, when our prehistoric ancestors lived. Maybe every few months there was a tiger trying to eat us; today, it may feel like there's a tiger out to get us each and every day. In PVT the dorsal vagal shut-down is seen as a system to ensure self-preservation. It's like a cap to control sympathetic activation and stop it from blowing up. When sympathetic activation due to trauma or chronic stress is ongoing over a longer time period or is too intense, dorsal vagal shut-down takes over to protect your body and being.

What's important to understand is that we are just as much under stress in dorsal vagal shut-down as we are in sympathetic activation. So even though we may seem quiet, controlled and calm on the outside, on the inside we are actually in constant survival mode. Some of us may be aware of this, but most of us aren't. The implications are severe, as we have learned that being in survival mode actually changes the way we view the world.[4] We begin to see danger when there is none, and even neutral faces are more likely to be perceived as angry. Our perception of physical stimuli changes, and we become more sensitive to pain. Energy and performance are reduced as the constant survival state drains our batteries. Digestion, rest and physical recovery may all be impaired. And last but not least, our cognitive performance and ability to connect are reduced.

We are affected on all levels of the being: physically, mentally and emotionally.

Before moving into the series of tools and practices, starting with exercises around breathing, let me help you understand the role of the vagus nerve in our stress responses in a simplified way. Our vagus nerve is the longest cranial nerve in the body and its purpose is to control involuntary functions of the parasympathetic nervous system, such as heart rate, digestion and immune system. A bit like a bouncer in front of a nightclub, who controls how many people enter the club depending on its capacity, our vagus nerve controls how we react to stress and helps up- or down-regulate the nervous system accordingly. When there is too much activity within the club, as in too many people (too much stress), the vagus nerve restricts new people from entering (sympathetic fight or flight response). Once things get a bit quieter inside and more people have left the club (coming back up the ladder), the vagus nerve allows for new people to enter (ventral vagal social engagement response).

This up- and down regulation of the nervous system happens naturally and unconsciously, in people with a strong vagal tone. For those affected by chronic stress and pain, or those suffering from trauma, this system is often distorted, and vagal tone is poor. Where other people can have an argument with their spouses or face a dangerous situation in traffic without consequences and can quickly recover, those with poor vagal tone cannot. Many more stress hormones are dumped than needed, and signals of safety and support are not being sent through. The purpose of the vagus nerve is to help you trigger that relaxation response and return to a sense of safety.

It is important to understand that working with the vagus nerve is about working directly with the body and its physiological responses. It is not about imagining or interpreting thoughts, ideas or behaviors. The main ways to directly affect the vagal tone and work on improving it are through working with the breath and working with touch. For this reason, the majority of the workbook focuses on these two modalities.

We will explore tools and techniques to help you better understand your vagal tone and how your personal stress bouncer is currently working. We will also show you effective tools to learn to self-regulate your nervous system. Most of the tools that will be introduced can be successfully used alone. Some can be even more effective with the help of a PVT professional. Since an important aspect of PVT is co-regulation and being able to receive cues of safety and support from others, ultimately our healing process needs to include finding a way back into safe interactions with others. For this reason, I will dedicate the last part of this workbook entirely to exploring social interactions and relations in PVT. There, you will learn more about how others can help you feel calm and relaxed through a process called co-regulation. Moving away from simply striving to survive on our own and returning to a longing to connect and perceiving the world as a safe place.

For many people suffering from anxiety, chronic stress, PTSD or C-PTSD, dissociation or depression, such a life and longing for connection may seem very far away. Others may even be perceived as the source of our problems and illnesses. As someone once said, "If you don't heal what hurt you, you will bleed on the people who didn't cut you." There is a lot of truth to this. Getting stitches might take longer than the actual cut, but depending on how deep the cut is, it might be the only way for it to heal properly and safely. Working with PVT is like getting stitches or using a scar cream for old wounds that haven't properly healed or left too big a scar. It's a framework for working with trauma through the body.

PART 2

Learning or Re-Learning to Self-Regulate

Self-regulation is the capacity to manage our internal experiences, such as our emotions, energy, thoughts and bodily reactions. Ideally, we learn to self-regulate in early childhood so that we are equipped for life and all the ups and downs that it can bring. Unfortunately, many of us don't, and those who have experienced trauma or are suffering from chronic stress or other psychological illnesses usually have an impaired self-regulation system. Remember the nightclub bouncer in the previous section? In this case he would let people in, even though the club is already at maximum capacity. So for most of us on our healing journeys, finding effective ways to regulate our thoughts, emotions and sensations is a first and important step.

We need to learn to come back to a place of calmness and grounding by learning to send signals of safety to our ANS. In this second part, we will do exactly this. You will be learning and trying out numerous tools to help you self-regulate by directly or indirectly working with the vagus nerve. The main modalities I will introduce here are working with your breath and working through physical touch. Remember to have your journal ready, a curious attitude and a beginner's mindset while you try out these tools and practices.

If at any point you are feeling overwhelmed, triggered, or even finding yourself going into a state of dissociation from the body, remember to seek the support of a professional or a person of trust. Maybe you can identify such a person right now. Just think of someone that you can call and ask for support, just in case you ever find yourself overwhelmed. By the way, we should all have such a person, whether we are going through this workbook or not.

In any such moments, try to regulate your breath (if you were breathing deeply, for example, reduce the depth a bit), stay or come back into your body, feel your body and specifically, feel the ground underneath you. You can also use a little stress ball or something you can fidget with if you are noticing a sense of overwhelm. These are just some general recommendations in case you are going through this workbook on your own. If you are a licensed professional working with clients or patients, surely you have your own repertoire of methods to support clients through difficult moments in sessions. Experiencing and successfully going through difficult moments often is part of the healing process. I know it's not easy. I have been there as well. I invite you to trust in your innate capacity to support yourself through difficult situations, and I trust in your discernment to reach out for support when you find you cannot handle a situation by yourself.

CHAPTER 1

Activating the Vagus Nerve Through Your Breath

Remember that your vagus nerve sends signals from the brain to the internal organs such as the heart, the lungs and even the gut. In many cases, such as an over activation of the sympathetic nervous system and an increased stress response, you will want to increase vagal tone and vagal activation. In these cases, the nervous system needs to be downregulated to help you return from activation and stress to relaxation and calmness. The first tools will specifically look at helping you move from sympathetic activation back into a ventral vagal social engagement.

1. Six Breaths Per Minute

Most adults take somewhere between 12 and 20 breaths per minute. That is one breath every 3 to 5 seconds. In this first tool, we are going to practice simply reducing the number of breaths per minute to slow down the overall breathing. I suggest for this practice to reduce the number of breaths to 6 per minute. If you start the practice and find yourself struggling with a shortage of air, increase the number of breaths per minute to 10 or 15 if needed. Most of us are so out of practice with this slower and usually deeper way of breathing that such an exercise can be challenging to begin. After 3 or 4 times, though, you will find things getting much easier. This is a guided practice. You may read the instructions below but I've gone ahead and made audio you can listen along to for a more seamless experience. You can download and listen to the audio version of these instructions by the scanning the QR code below. Or you can get access them at this url: *https://bit.ly/ptmadesimple*

Take about 3 to 5 minutes for this practice. You can really do this anywhere; a quiet space, ideally for yourself and where you feel safe, is best. If you have a stopwatch for this practice, that is even better.

- Begin by finding yourself a comfortable seat in a chair or on the ground, supported by some cushions. You want to be comfortable, but not so comfortable that you run the risk of falling asleep.

- Ensure that your spine is straight, gently raise the shoulder up and back, relax your head, neck and any tension in the face, especially around the jaw.

- Check in with your body and if there is any discomfort, make any final adjustments. Then try to stay still for the duration of the practice.

- Simply begin by paying attention to your breath. Just notice the rhythm and speed of your natural breath. You may notice that you are breathing a bit shallow or fast.

- Set a one-minute timer on your stopwatch or phone. Start it and begin counting the number of breaths you take until one minute is up. One breath is one full inhale and one full exhale.

- How many breaths did you take in one minute?

- Now set that timer again, and reduce the amount of breaths you take in that one minute by half. If you took 24 breaths in one minute before, take 12 now. It doesn't need to be 100% exact. The point is to slow your breathing drastically.

- See if you can continue this practice until you can reduce the number of breaths you take in one minute to 6. This would mean taking 10 seconds for every complete breath in and out.

- If there is too much strain, dizziness or you begin feeling lightheaded, stop reducing the number of breaths and breathe naturally. It's important to remember as we breathe slower, we usually breathe deeper, meaning we breathe out more carbon dioxide than we can produce. This can create dizziness at first but will pass with time and especially with practice.

- Breathe normally to end the practice and just observe how you feel. You can journal any insights, if you like.

If the nervous system is under stress, you find your heart racing, muscles tensing and the body being flooded with stress hormones. This sort of practice can really help calm you and go back from sympathetic activation to ventral vagal activation.

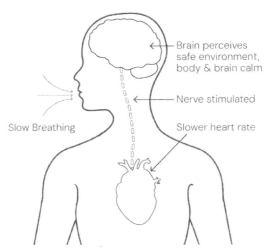

23

2. Deep Belly Breathing

Most people are shallow or upper-chest breathers. They inhale through the nose and mouth, keep the air in the chest, and never fully allow the air to expand to the diaphragm and the belly. Shallow breathing does not provide your body and mind with sufficient fresh oxygen and can negatively impact your energy level, mental clarity and concentration.[5] If you think back to PVT and the ladder of stress responses introduced by Deb Dana, shallow breathing is part of the sympathetic stress response. Shallow breathing can be a consequence of perceived danger, putting the body in fight or flight. Logically, to dissolve this, the answer is slow and deep abdominal breathing, which activates the vagus nerve and parasympathetic nervous system.

Deep abdominal breathing is something that most of us have never properly learned and are not generally practicing. Yet, it is such an easy practice to do on your own, no matter where you are. At this time, it is important to note that if you are suffering from trauma, PTSD or c-PTSD, deep abdominal breathing may potentially trigger a stress response. For people suffering from these conditions, the body is often not perceived as a safe space, so coming back into and connecting with the body through deep breathing can actually magnify not feeling safe or feeling anxious. In these cases, you may need to learn through other, softer methods and with the help of support, that feeling and tuning into the body is safe. Just taking fewer breaths per minute (while counting) or practicing equal breathing might be more accessible, as there is also a mental task involved in these practices.

The following practice can also be done alongside a guided audio recording. You may read the instructions below but I've gone ahead and made audio you can listen along to for a more seamless experience.

You can download and listen to the audio version of these instructions by the scanning the QR code below.

Or you can get access them at this url: *https://bit.ly/ptmadesimple*

Take 5 to 7 minutes for this practice and find a place where you can comfortably sit or even lie down.

- Choose your position: Stand, sit, or lie down (lying down is best for beginners prone to dizziness, with pillows under head and knees).

- Adjust your posture: Bring shoulders up and back, open the chest, and relax tension in the face, arms, and legs.

- Relax the jaw and eyes. If comfortable and safe, close your eyes. Otherwise, focus on a point on the ceiling or wall.

- Start breathing naturally, noticing how the air enters through your nose, travels down your throat and fills your chest.

- Take deep exhalations through the mouth, possibly sighing to aid relaxation.

- Inhale deeper through the nose, filling the chest and lungs, then filling the belly with air.

- Place one hand on the chest and one on the belly to feel the rise and fall of breath.

- Allow the belly to expand naturally as it fills with air.

- Exhale through the mouth by pursing lips, starting with the belly and gently squeezing abdominal muscles to release all air.

- Gently squeeze your abdominal muscles to help you release all the air. It may take a few practice rounds in order to breathe naturally in this way. The following image visualizes this practice:

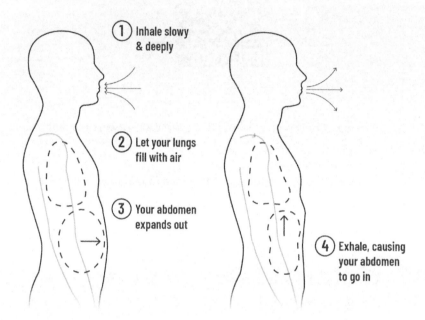

1. Inhale slowy & deeply
2. Let your lungs fill with air
3. Your abdomen expands out
4. Exhale, causing your abdomen to go in

3. Equal Breathing

A breathing practice you will find in many yoga classes or when searching the internet for practices to activate the vagus nerve through your breath is equal or square breathing. It's named in this way for its balanced approach to inhaling, holding, exhaling and holding, which helps reduce blood pressure and bring a sense of calm almost instantly.[6] It works similarly to the previous breathing practices, activating the vagus nerve and initiating the activation of the parasympathetic nervous system.

- Before we begin, take a moment to relax. Stretch out, move a bit, whatever helps release any tension in your body. Find a comfortable spot, whether sitting in a chair with your back straight or lying down—it's about being relaxed yet alert.

- Now, here's how it works: Inhale slowly, counting to 4 in your mind. Hold your breath for another count of 4. Then, exhale slowly to the count of 4. Lastly, hold your breath again for 4 counts. This completes one round.

- Try to flow from one round to the next seamlessly. At first, it may feel a bit challenging to hold your breath for those few seconds without feeling uneasy. If it feels too uncomfortable or brings up anxiety, it's okay to skip the breath holds for now. You can always come back to them when you feel more comfortable.

- As you breathe, the rhythm will look like this:
  Inhale - 1 - 2 - 3 - 4
  Hold - 1 - 2 - 3 - 4
  Exhale - 1 - 2 - 3 - 4
  Hold - 1 - 2 - 3 - 4

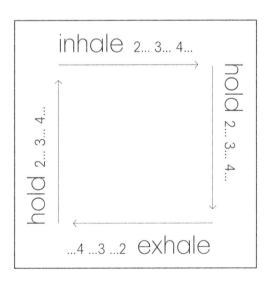

Try practicing this for about 3 to 10 minutes whenever you have a moment. Afterward, take some time to reflect on how you feel. It's a simple practice, but it can really help ground you and bring some peace into your day. Remember, the most important thing is to listen to your body and only do what feels comfortable and calming for you.

4. Breathing and Heart Rate Variability

Heart rate variability is the variation in time between heartbeats. A healthy person's heart does not always beat at the same rhythm. When things upset us in everyday life, we get excited, agitated or even angry. Our heart rates increase, adjusting our bodies internally to what is happening on the outside. Then, when the reason for our excitement or upset passes, our heart rates should decrease again naturally and relatively quickly. A high heart rate variability is linked to overall health.

Studies suggest that there is even a link between low heart rate variability and psychiatric illnesses such as depression, substance abuse and schizophrenia.[7] A low heart rate variability can come with future health problems, as your body is less capable of physically handling challenging situations. Often, people with higher resting heart rates have lower heart rate variability. While this is going a bit off-topic, I would like to mention at this point that your heart rate variability can be naturally increased through regular exercise, a healthy diet, plenty of water and sleep, and reducing alcohol and stress. The regular health recommendations, as you can see. Breathing slower, deep belly breathing, and square breathing all seem to have a positive effect on heart rate variability.

Resonant or coherent breathing is currently the most widely spread breathing technique that has a direct influence on your heart rate variability. It is similar to the first practice in this workbook, as our speed of breathing is radically decreased.

For the best experience, listen to the audio recording accessible by scanning the following QR code or by using this url: *https://bit.ly/ptmadesimple*

If you cannot listen to the audio, see if you can find yourself a pacemaker online that signals you when to breathe in and out. There are many recordings out there nowadays, most playing some kind of music or sounds that signal you to inhale as the notes rise and out as they fall.

- Begin by finding yourself a comfortable place to stand or sit. Take a deep breath in through your nose, and then fully exhale through the mouth. Do this a couple of times to prepare yourself for the practice.

- See if you can relax the body a bit more, or shake out any tension. If it is available for you, close your eyes or at least partially close them, looking at a non-moving object on the ground or the wall in front of you.

- Start to breathe regularly and listen for the cues of the pacemaker. Inhale as the music rises, and exhale as it falls.

- Simply follow the music to the best of your ability. If your breathing is a bit off at times, that's fine. Just come back to following the rhythm when you can.

- Continue this practice for the duration of the music.

- Finish the exercise by breathing naturally at your own rhythm. Notice how your body and mind feels. Notice any sense of calm and relaxation.

5. Synchronized Breath

Many people track their heart rate variability using smartwatches or apps now. If you have such an app or device, you can also begin to explore tracking your heart rate variability for a week. It is best to take a measurement first in the morning after you wake up. You may have also heard of biofeedback, which, over time, can help you learn to control involuntary bodily functions such as your heart rate and breathing. Usually this is done in a lab or clinic, but there are also devices for your personal tracking at home. As you might imagine, being able to have more control over involuntary bodily functions can be very helpful in cases of anxiety or chronic pain. It can be really empowering when you learn over time that, with practice, you do not have to be at the mercy of all of your bodily symptoms and often have more control than you think.

At this time, I would like to invite you to do a short walking meditation that is synchronized with your breath. Ideally, you can go for a little walk outside in a park or in nature, where there are few distractions. If you don't have this possibility or don't want to go outside, do this practice in the largest room of your house. If it's warm enough and safe, take off your shoes and socks and do this barefoot. You can fold your hands in front of you, resting on your belly or behind your back. Take a moment to pause and feel within before you start. In this practice, you will be invited to walk much slower than usual. There is no rush to go or get anywhere. The practice should last at least 5 or 10 minutes.

You will begin walking by lifting the right foot and placing it just a few centimeters or inches in front of you. As you lift and move your right foot, inhale. Then continue by lifting and moving your left foot just a few centimeters or inches to the front. As you move your left foot, exhale. This is your rhythm; this is all you do. Inhale, moving the right foot; exhale, moving the left foot. Move in a circle around the room, or back and forth if the room is not very wide. Keep your eyes focused on the ground in front of you and your attention directed on the walking and the breathing. See if you can really synchronize breathing and taking slow, small steps.

If you are outside, let go of the idea of how this may look or what others may think. Ideally, you can practice this in a not-so-busy place where you will be undisturbed. Enjoy the walking meditation and journal afterward about how you felt!

6. "Ha" Breathing

Most of the breathing practices described here support the down-regulation of the nervous system. With your breath, you aim to help yourself out of the sympathetic stress response and back into ventral vagal social engagement. You might not feel fully ready to dive back into social engagement after your body feels really stressed, but at least you are likely to experience yourself more calm and relaxed. Now, what about situations when someone is stuck in dorsal vagal shut-down?

You may remember from *Part 1* and Deb Dana's ladder that this nervous system response is at the bottom of said ladder. When the sympathetic activation is ongoing or is too intense, dorsal vagal shut-down takes over to protect you. A person with this response may feel or even look frozen and paralyzed. Heart rate and blood pressure decrease. Breathing becomes more shallow, and someone may emotionally detach. If you work with clients, you know what this can look like. In some cases, though, this is not visible at all. People who have been spending so much time in dorsal and ventral shut-down may have found ways to mask the fact that they are actually in a permanent survival mode. And most of the time, people don't even know this themselves.

Depending on your experience and sensitivity, you may feel generally unwell, tense or anxious yourself being around someone with such a response. It may be as though before you met them, everything was fine, but after you have spent five minutes in their presence your nervous system may react with signs of stress and tension. We will speak more about this in the last part on co-regulation. It's important to differentiate if feeling stressed or tense has other sources, such as if the person did something that upsets you or generally triggers you. This is not what I mean here. It's about unconsciously information about another's nervous system when words don't match your perceptions. This is something that can be learned over time, but of course, some people have easier access to this kind of information than others.

So let me share an easy practice with you that will help you or your clients up-regulate your nervous system in case someone is stuck in dorsal-ventral shutdown and needs to mobilize themselves. The practice is very simple and, as you may imagine, a bit more active. You can begin by taking a few deep breaths in and out, freeing the body of any unnecessary tension, and shaking it out if needed. It's best to do this practice standing. Now take a deep inhale through the nose, filling the lungs and chest with air, then exhale through the mouth, making a "ha" sound. Each round of inhale and exhale should take you around 3 to 6 seconds. Repeat this about 10 to 20 times, and you may notice your body getting more energized as it and the brain are supplied with extra oxygen. As you do this practice more often, you can increase the number of repetitions. It is important to remember, as you try to up-regulate the nervous system in this way, to always move gradually and without force. So it's better to move slower with fewer repetitions to begin, and then increase speed and the number of repetitions.

How do you feel after this exercise? If you are finding yourself very lethargic, without energy or motivation, and somehow feeling stuck, this practice can help you out of that. Do note that you may enter into sympathetic activation as a result, and if this activation is overwhelming for you, you may go back into dorsal shut-down.

Making your way back into ventral vagal social engagement is a process that, depending on your condition, may take time and may require the support of a professional. In most cases, whatever brought you to the shutdown in the first place needs to be safely experienced and felt in order to move out of the shut-down response. Also, be compassionate with yourself if you find yourself moving up the nervous system response ladder introduced in *Part 1.*

7. Mindfulness Meditation on Your Breath

Practicing mindfulness meditation with a focus on the breath can deeply align with PVT, offering a simple way to regulate the ANS and promote a sense of safety and well-being.[8] Just like in slow or deep belly breathing, through mindful breathing you stimulate the vagus nerve, and encourage a shift of your nervous systems into the rest and digest. Now what exactly is mindful breathing, and how does it work? Mindful breathing is exactly what the name implies: breathing mindfully while also becoming aware of any bodily sensations. It is breathing while becoming aware of any tension, pain or discomfort in the body. There is no specific way to breathe. You are simply being invited to breathe with aware-ness, to watch your breath and how it moves in and out, and how the body feels while you breathe in this mindful way. You are invited to notice any areas of tension in the body, and see if you can ease up the tension simply by becoming aware or redirecting your breath.

Here is a guided mindfulness meditation that you can also listen to through the audio recording by scanning the following QR code, or by using this url: *https://bit.ly/ptmadesimple*

- Begin by finding a quiet and comfortable place where you can sit or lie down without distractions. Close your eyes gently, and allow yourself to settle into a relaxed posture. Take a few moments to notice the support beneath you—the ground or chair—and consciously release any tension you may be holding in your body.

- Start by bringing your awareness to your breath. Feel the natural rhythm of your breath without trying to control it. Notice the gentle rise and fall of your chest and abdomen with each inhale and exhale. Pay attention to the sensations of the air as it enters through your nostrils and fills your lungs, as well as the feeling of release as you exhale.

- As you continue to breathe, bring a sense of curiosity and openness to the experience. Allow your breath to be your anchor to the present moment, grounding you in the here and now. If your mind starts to wander—as it naturally does—gently guide your attention back to the sensations of your breath. This practice is not about suppressing thoughts, but rather gently redirecting your focus each time you notice distraction.

- How are you doing right now?

- Ensure that this practice is still available for you and that you are alert and awake enough to continue. Sometimes this form of mindful breathing or being mindful in general can be extremely tiring and put us right to sleep. The reason is that we are not used to slowing down in this way, or there may also be some form of internal defense mechanism at play. Somehow, you may not be ready for this practice yet.

- If you encounter any difficult emotions or sensations during this practice—such as anxiety, restlessness, or discomfort—approach with gentle acceptance. Allow these to exist without judgment, knowing that your breath and presence can provide a supportive container for whatever arises.

- Continue this practice for several minutes, gradually extending the duration if it feels comfortable. As you near the end of your practice, take a moment to reflect on how you feel. Notice any shifts in your mood, energy or sense of calmness compared to when you began.

- To conclude, bring your attention back to your surroundings. Wiggle your fingers and toes, gently stretch your body if needed, and open your eyes when you're ready.

Incorporating mindful breathing into your daily routine can serve as a powerful tool for self-care and emotional regulation, aligning with the principles of PVT. Regular practice can help you cultivate resilience, enhance your ability to cope with stress, and foster a deeper connection with your inner sense of peace and well-being.

8. Exhaling Bodily Tension

If you did the previous practice, or any of the other exercises, and discovered tension in your body or if difficult thoughts or emotions arise, here is another practice that can help you navigate this. The assumption of PVT is that regulation of the nervous system is not happening in a way that supports homeostasis in the being, meaning up- and down-regulation of the nervous system (a calming or energizing of the body) is not happening the way it should. Whether this is because it was never learned, falsely learned or due to a one-time or a series of traumatic events experienced, this doesn't matter so much. Remember, with PVT it is not about the story of what happened to you, but about how you are still experiencing what happened to you in your body and about the fact that you are still experiencing limitations today. More on this in the parts about trauma.

All of us experience tensions in the body, mind and emotions at times that are more or less severe. Many people like you or the clients you are working with are experiencing so much tension that builds up and up over time. When someone with this much built-up tension begins to feel it in their body, the perceived phenomena can be very intense. Yet, the only way to move out of this way of tension is to move it. To experience it and experience yourself while feeling it.

If you were hoping that it would just go away one day, I'm afraid I do not have good news for you. The good news I do share, though, is that you have a hidden superpower with you at all times! You have your breath. Personally, I wish someone would have told or shown me how I could use my breath to regulate these tensions in my body while I was growing up. I hear clients sharing similar things once they have discovered the power of their own breath for controlling and moving inner tension. You can do this practice during any of the other exercises, specifically during the mindfulness meditation. Basically, any time you discover tensions in your physical body, in your mind or through your emotions, give this technique a try.

What you are going to do when you notice the tension in your body, mind or emotions, is to gently redirect your breath there. You can take a bit of a deeper inhale, and during this inhale redirect your attention and breath on the pain. Say that your back hurts for example. You can gently bring your awareness there when you breathe in. It is as if you are sending your breath directly to the part that feels painful. Let it hang out there for one or two seconds, then breathe out and imagine that the pain is leaving the body with the exhale. Do this for some minutes, depending on the severity of the physical pain.

You can even imagine breathing certain qualities of healing, relaxation and support into the areas of pain. While you are doing all this, you are focused on the breath and where it is redirected in your body, but you are also trying to watch and be aware of the entire experience. This exercise can be very powerful, and you may literally experience pain leaving your body. This does take some practice of course and there is a possibility that initially the perceived pain worsens for a few minutes. Usually this passes as you continue with the practice, and with imagining releasing the tension or pain on the exhalation. Please note that this can also work with emotions and thoughts, but if you find the intensity through redirecting your breath in this way too high, please stop.

If you don't believe this can work, just remember the last time you really hurt yourself physically, and how you may have increased and deepened your breath, trying to breathe the pain away or out. At least this is my experience.

9. Dissolving Bodily Tension

Another very similar technique to the last that I would like to mention at this point is not exhaling the tension, but rather dissolving it. So instead of inhaling into the tension and exhaling it out of your body, you would inhale into the tension, keep your breath there for some time, and imagine it slowly dissolving the tension, pain or discomfort. It's like inhaling, redirecting your breath to any pain or tension, and then holding your breath there for a few seconds, letting it linger there for a bit. You can visually imagine a dissolution of the perceived discomfort, seeing it disappear before your eyes. When inhaling, you can imagine your breath being charged with love, softness and healing power, which then come to rest in the area of tension and dissolve them. This practice may be a bit harder for the mind to grasp, but why not give it a try? Again, if you are finding that the discomfort and tensions become much stronger, even unbearable, as you are redirecting your breath and attention in this way, leave this practice for later and/or under the guidance of a licensed professional.

10. Alternate Nostril Breathing

For the Yogis, there is a whole science behind working with the breath for physical, mental and emotional well-being called *Pranayama*. Many of the breathing practices mentioned here are also typical yogic practices. Pranayama is aimed at creating more harmony between body and mind, so please be wary if you do not feel ready to come back into your body in this way quite yet. One of my personal favorites when it comes to yogic breathing practices that have a calming effect, helping to clear the mind and even emotions, is alternate nostril breathing, also known as *Nadi Shodhana*. It is a technique that involves breathing through one nostril at a time while using the fingers to block and alternate between them. This practice is deeply connected to PVT as it also activates the vagus nerve, igniting a parasympathetic nervous system response and helping to calm the body. Here is how you can practice on your own. The following practice can also be done using the guided audio created for it.

You can access it by scanning the following QR code or using this link: *https://bit.ly/ptmadesimple*

- Prepare yourself by finding a comfortable seated position on the floor or on a chair, with the spine straight and shoulders up and back. Take three full ventilation breaths, fully inhaling through the nose and filling your chest and lungs with air, then exhale deeply through the mouth while you bend forward to release all the air. Do this again a few times and make a sound on the exhalation for a better release of tension.

- Assume the following hand position with your fingers: With your right hand, bring your index and middle fingers to rest between your eyebrows. For the following practice, you are going to use your thumb to close your right nostril and your ring finger or pinky to close your left nostril. To close one nostril, you simply press your finger on the side of that nostril from the outside. You will alternate between closing the right and left nostril, and not close both nostrils at the same time. Rest your left hand comfortably on your left knee or thigh.

- Now, begin the practice by closing the right nostril. Gently press your right thumb against your right nostril, closing it off completely. Then inhale deeply and slowly through the left nostril. Focus on the sensation of the breath entering your body.

- Continue by switching sides and closing your left nostril with your ring or pinky finger, releasing your right nostril, and simultaneously exhaling slowly and completely through the right nostril.

- Continue by inhaling through the right nostril while keeping your left nostril closed. Inhale slowly and deeply through your right nostril.

- Switch sides again and close your right nostril with your thumb, release your left nostril, and exhale slowly and completely through your left nostril.

- Repeat and continue this pattern, inhaling through the nostril that you just exhaled from and exhaling through the opposite nostril. Maintain a smooth and steady breath, focusing on the rhythm and sensation of the air moving through each nostril.

- If you find your nose blocked or running, feel free to interrupt to blow your nose. Also, don't get caught up on any sounds you might be making as you are inhaling, and see if you can allow air through, even if the sinuses are a bit blocked. This practice can be great for slightly blocked sinuses and can even help with the treatment of sinusitis over time. If your sinuses are acutely and completely blocked, do not practice Nadi Shodhana.

- Conclude the practice after several rounds, or typically 5–10 minutes. Release your hand from your face and return to normal breathing. Take a moment to observe any changes in your mental state, emotional well-being, or physical sensations.

Alternate nostril breathing is believed to balance the activity of the left and right hemispheres of the brain and stimulate the vagus nerve. Practicing alternate nostril breathing can increase vagal tone over time, helping you modulate your stress response more flexibly.[9] Start with a few minutes and gradually increase the duration as you become more comfortable with the technique.

11. Ujjayi Breathing

In the first part of this book, you are really being introduced to the best of the best breathing techniques that yogis have been practicing for thousands of years. We will leave you with two more practices that are a little bit more specific, as they require the constriction of some additional muscles while breathing. First, let's speak about Ujjayi pranayama, often referred to as "victorious breath" or "ocean breath." In this practice, you will need to gently constrict the muscles in the back of the throat to create a soft whispering sound during both inhalation and exhalation. The purpose of this practice is to deepen concentration, calm the mind, and regulate the flow of prana or life force energy, throughout the body. And of course, as you may imagine, Ujjayi pranayama activates the vagus nerve. Here is how you can practice: Read the instructions below or listen to the guided audio for this exercise by scanning the following QR code or accessing via this url: *https://bit.ly/ptmadesimple*

- As in all meditations and breathing practices, find yourself in a comfortable seated position with your spine straight, bringing the shoulders up and back. You can sit cross-legged on the floor or on a chair with your feet flat on the ground. If it is available for you, gently close your eyes to turn your focus inward. If not, just pick a point on the floor or wall in front of you.

- Take a few deep breaths to settle in and release any tension from your body. Allow everything to settle and invite a sense of relaxation.

- Begin by inhaling deeply and slowly through your nose. Feel the air entering your nostrils, filling your lungs, and expanding your chest and abdomen.

- As you exhale through your nose, gently constrict the muscles at the back of your throat. If you are unsure how to contract these muscles, imagine fogging up a mirror with your breath. This gentle constriction creates a soft, whispering sound, like wind through the trees.

- Continue inhaling deeply through your nose, maintaining the slight constriction at the back of your throat. Feel the breath moving smoothly and effortlessly.

- See if you can make your inhalations and exhalations of equal duration. This helps to balance the flow of energy and maintain a steady rhythm.

- As you continue with this technique, bring your awareness to the sound and sensation of your breath. Notice how the whispering sound reverberates in your throat and resonates throughout your body.

- Practice for several minutes, gradually increasing the duration as you become more comfortable with the technique. As a beginner, it's best to start with 5 minutes per day and gradually increase the duration over time.

- Finish the practice by releasing the contraction in the throat and returning to natural breathing. Take a moment to notice your mental state, any physical sensations, or your overall sense of well-being after the exercise.

Regular practice of Ujjayi pranayama can help to enhance concentration, reduce stress and promote relaxation. It also helps to develop greater awareness of the breath and its connection to our inner state of being.

12. Sitali and Sitkari Pranayama

Last but not least let me share with you two cooling breathing practices. These might not just come in handy to help you calm down and relax, but can also be effectively used when you are in a very hot environment, as they help cool the body temperature. They may also create some laughter and can be another beautiful practice to do with a friend or partner.

I will explain both practices briefly. You are invited to simply try each practice for a few minutes to begin. Since both exercises may require a bit of practice, give them a try and pick the one that resonates most.

Sitali Pranayama:

- Roll your tongue into a "U" shape, sticking it slightly out of your mouth.

- Inhale deeply and slowly through your rolled tongue, feel the coolness of the breath as it enters your mouth.

- Close your mouth and exhale slowly and completely through your nose.

- Repeat this process for several rounds, focusing on the cooling sensation of the breath and the rhythmic pattern of inhalation and exhalation.

- Note: Some people are not able to roll their tongue. If this is the case for you, practice sitkari pranayama.

Sitkari Pranayama:

- Close your lips gently, keeping your teeth slightly apart.

- Inhale deeply and slowly through your teeth, feeling the cool air passing over your tongue and into your mouth.

- Close your mouth and exhale slowly and completely through your nose.

- Continue this practice for several rounds, maintaining awareness of the cooling effect and the sound of the breath passing through your teeth.

- Please note: For some people, this may create sensitivity in the teeth. If this is the case for you, see if you prefer Sitali pranayama.

Both techniques involve conscious control of the breath, therefore stimulating the vagus nerve. Incorporating these cooling pranayama techniques into the day can be supportive with stress reduction, enhance vagal tone, and promote a sense of inner calm and balance. As these practices may take some getting used to, adjust the time of the exercise to your individual needs. As we continue to move through this workbook, you will be invited more and more into adapting the exercises in a way that fits you best.

A big part of self-regulation and healing is learning to become more aware of and listen to the cues of the body. Our bodies often signal to us clearly about what we need and what we don't, it's just that we were never taught how to listen or we simply forgot. Always listen to your body, read and interpret the cues and then see if the bodily cue is appropriate for the specific situation. If the bodily reaction seems quite strong or even too extreme for a specific situation, chances are something else is at play. If you feel ready, then this is your possibility for deeper healing. If not, that's ok too. There will be more opportunities. Listening in with openness and curiosity as you try all of these practices and adjusting them to your needs is most important.

13. Chanting, Humming or Gargling

As we come to the end of this first chapter, in which you were introduced to many tools to help you activate your vagus nerve through your breath, let's mention a few more methods that are not directly linked to your breath but are simple ways to activate your parasympathetic nervous system without touch.

First chanting the universal sound "Om" or a simple humming. When you chant and hum, you are constantly extending your exhalations. This and the vibrations created in the neck area stimulate the vagus nerve and therefore activate the parasympathetic nervous system. It's so simple, and you might feel silly doing it, but the next time you are in your car on your way to work to give an important presentation, give these techniques a try. You are likely to feel a mix of feeling slightly energized, and calm and relaxed. Plus, it's a great way to warm up your voice before public speaking. For many years, I also taught yoga and meditation, sometimes in front of 60 to 70 people. Every morning on my way to class, I would hum and do a little singing practice. After the 5-minute walk, I would feel more awake and clear-headed, while also feeling very calm. Students also appreciated the gentle and warmed-up voice.

Another very simple but powerful method to strengthen the vagal tone is through the simple gargling of water. It is recommended that you do this practice twice a day for up to 30 seconds. You could integrate this into your morning routine after you have brushed your teeth. You can use plain, lukewarm water for this. Make sure you have removed all the toothpaste from your mouth before you begin to gargle. Once you have gotten comfortable gargling, you can begin to practice more vigorously, making loud sounds. If you invite your partner into this practice, you may find a fun, playful morning routine that not only helps you start the day with ease but also feel more connected to each other.

In this first chapter of *Part 1* of the workbook, you were being introduced to many different practices of working with your breath to down- and up-regulate your nervous system and activate your vagus nerve. Many of the practices were similar at the core, all with different nuances though. You may have found some practices work better for you than others. Some may have made you feel safe and relaxed; others may have created a sense of tension and maybe even anxiety.

Trust the wisdom of your body and practice, and repeat those practices that feel most aligned and supportive at this time. If a practice did not work for you, it is perfectly okay to have skipped it for now, but be sure to mark it somehow so you can come back and try it again later. Healing is really a gradual process, and something that we may not be ready for today could be something of great support in a few weeks or months. From my experience, the healing process can even be a bit mysterious at times, and things that you were struggling with at some point may become your preferred tool or practice in the future.

CHAPTER 2

Activating the Vagus Nerve Through Touch

L et's continue this exploration of ways in which you can learn or re-learn to regulate your own nervous system. In this next chapter, we will focus on tools related to touch. Remember that the vagus nerve helps modulate between different nervous system responses and that the stronger the vagal tone, the better the capacity to regulate stress.[10] Where the last chapter focused on the vagus nerve activation and down- as well as up-regulation of the nervous system through using your breath, this chapter will focus entirely on practices that work with touch. The tools in this chapter and the last follow no specific order in terms of how and when they should be used. It's totally up to you, or your clients, which tools to begin working with.

The tools I will mention here are ones you can try out yourself. They are general tools that are intended to be available to everyone, with or without the support of a licensed professional. I will clearly mark which tools can activate your parasympathetic nervous system, helping you calm and relax, and which can activate your sympathetic nervous system, ideally helping you get out of a parasympathetic collapse or freeze response. Of course, different practices may personally affect you differently. Therefore, it is recommended to go on with care and gentleness, and when in doubt, skip a practice and come back to it later.

If you find any practice to be exceptionally difficult or find yourself feeling very uncomfortable or even overwhelmed during a practice, consider working with a specialist experienced in trauma work. When integrating the body into the healing process, there should be no sense of pushing or performing. It was your body that protected you from overwhelm and exhaustion through lasting sympathetic activation in the first place. Trust in the capacity of your body to help you out of this again. Read and re-read the following questions for contemplation, and let them invite you into a deeper sense of trust and confidence. What if the body actually had the same innate wisdom to help you out of the stress and trauma response that it initiated in the first place?

What if your body had much more wisdom than you thought? What if it was actually smarter than the mind, from which any sense of pushing and performing would originate? We will continue to explore this, especially in the next chapters on trauma and co-regulation. As you move through this chapter, see which practices naturally resonate with you. You can even ask your body if a specific practice feels aligned and appropriate at a given moment. You can ask the same question to your mind to see if it thinks that a practice is a good idea. See what arises and where mind and body differ. Always have your journal ready and capture any feelings, thoughts or insights.

1. Localizing the Vagus Nerve

Since in this chapter we will activate the vagus nerve through touch, let's begin by exploring the longest cranial nerve and its pathways a bit more. Take a look at the graphic below to understand the different pathways of the vagus nerve. As you can see, the vagus nerve pathways run between the brain and many different parts of the body, carrying signals mostly from the brain to the body, and in some instances from the body to the brain.

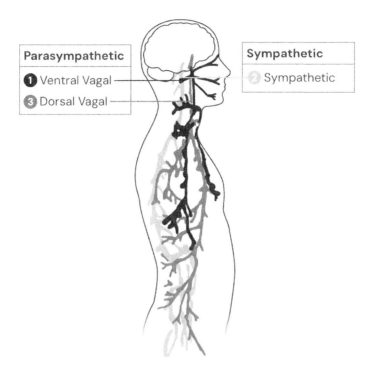

The different pathways of the nerve are generally responsible for the different nervous system responses.

1. The ventral vagal pathway is part of the parasympathetic nervous system response that is linked to nerves which control the face, neck, throat and inner ear.

2. The vagus nerve pathway that is linked to the sympathetic response runs down the back alongside the spine.

3. The dorsal vagal pathway that is linked to the shut-down response branches out into different areas of the torso and into different organs.

Notice that at the level of the head and neck, vagus nerve branches are found in a similar location before following the three mainly distinct pathways mentioned above. Anatomically and physiologically, it gets a lot more complex than this, but this is a workbook to be applied and not a medical textbook. The intention of sharing this image and the vagus nerve pathways is to give you some first ideas of how you can work with touch to activate this nerve.

Before we move into the different practices involving touch, take a moment to visualize these pathways before your inner eye. You can do this practice anywhere you feel comfortable and safe, having a few moments to yourself.

- Begin by imagining the ventral vagal pathway that runs through your face, throat and chest. You can simply bring your attention to the areas, and let it wander from one area to the next. Ideally you can have your eyes closed, but if this is not available for you, just look down at the ground or floor without focusing on any specific point. Imagine this pathway for one minute.

- Continue on with imagining the sympathetic activation of the vagus nerve that runs along your spinal cord. Just bring your attention to your spine and allow it to wander up and down it. Do this again for one minute.

- Lastly, bring your attention to the heart, diaphragm and gut. Let it wander through these organs. This can connect you to the dorsal vagal pathway linked to the shut-down response. Again, leave your attention on these areas for one minute.

I know that such a practice can be a bit tricky to begin with. Having a better understanding of what parts of the body are linked to what nervous system response can help you understand why we will touch the different areas of the body. Plus, we are generally strengthening the mind-body connection, and in this way better understanding over time the reactions of the body and how these may be linked to phenomena of the mind.

At the end of this practice, journal any insights or anything else that may have arisen during the exercise. Depending on your capacity to imagine and feel inside the body, you may perceive a lot of nothing. If you have ever experienced any trauma, difficult life events and/or stored emotions, such a practice may actually bring up difficult or painful memories. As with all the practices, take good care and move at your own speed. Seek support if you feel you need it, are finding yourself overwhelmed, or have something come up (like a difficult, painful or even traumatic memory).

2. Massaging the Ears

Let's begin to explore tools related to touch that activate the ventral vagal pathway, encouraging the sending of signs of safety and relaxation to the body. This will be needed, especially if you are finding yourself in sympathetic activation and fight or flight mode. Similarly, if you are finding yourself triggered and stressed as a result of any of the practices in this workbook, the following technique can activate the vagus nerve, helping you to down regulate the nervous system. Down-regulation is meant as the shift from sympathetic to parasympathetic (ventral vagal) activation. The first method we will explore in this chapter is the massaging of the ears. Allocate about 10 minutes for this practice.

- Choose a quiet, comfortable space to sit or stand. Using a mirror can help you better locate the massage points.

- Start by taking a few deep breaths, and ease any tension in your jaw by gently opening and closing your mouth as if you are yawning.

- Before you begin the massage, assess the tightness and flexibility of your ears by gently pulling on them. Repeat this assessment after the massage to see if anything changes.

- Refer to the illustrations below to identify the three massage points on the ear. Start with the first point shown on the left in the image. Massage this point in each ear for 1 to 2 minutes, adjusting the duration based on comfort. Focus on circular motions and gentle pressure rather than applying force. Alternate between ears, taking brief pauses between each pressure point.

- **Point 1:** Locate the small hollow above the ear canal, just above the ridge.

- **Point 2:** Find this point toward the rear of the ear canal.

- **Point 3:** Stretch the ear backwards, then downwards, and finally upwards, gently pulling and massaging the skin around the ear.

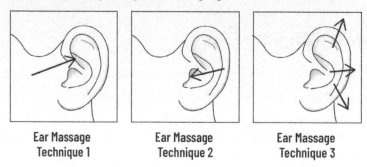

Ear Massage Technique 1   Ear Massage Technique 2   Ear Massage Technique 3

- When you finish massaging each point for a few minutes, reassess the tightness and flexibility of your ears by gently pulling on them. What has changed?

- Journal any insights. What was your favorite/least favorite massage point?

3. Massaging the Throat

Next, let's explore a practice to stimulate the vagus nerve manually that I personally find quite pleasurable. For the following practices in general, find yourself a comfortable and quiet spot to sit where you can be undisturbed for the duration of the practice. I know our busy lives can make it difficult to find such a place, especially if you are raising small children. I have worked with many moms and would always suggest to them to search for a quiet spot at least to begin. Many would respond that they simply do not have such a space, as their children don't even give them 5 minutes of privacy in the bathroom. Of course, if it's nearly impossible for you to find such a space because of whatever reason, this practice can be done anywhere (on a public bus, in the kitchen during dinner, on your bed before going to sleep, and so on).

Just to begin, as you are still strengthening your mind-body connection, it is helpful to do these practices without distraction and with focus. For many moms I've worked with, simply not having the space or time to do such a short exercise of less than five minutes often also had to do with them not being able to ask others, such as their partners, for help and giving up the responsibility for their children to someone else. Of course, this all depends on the age of the child, but I have seen this be a determining factor in the development of burnout in new moms. Without going off-topic here, the point is, if you do not have 5 minutes to yourself to do such a practice, I recommend seeing if you can make adjustments in your external environment.

Once you have your comfortable and quiet spot, take a few breaths and loosen your jaw by opening your mouth. You can also stick your tongue out and move it around for just a few seconds. Then do a slight stretching of the neck from side to side, bringing each ear to the respective shoulder, and turn your head from side to side. Bring the shoulders up and back, and then place your middle finger on your tragus. The tragus is the fleshy prominence at the front of the external opening of the ear, and right behind it is the entrance of the ear canal. Place both middle fingers on each tragus and, using your index finger, gently begin to massage the area behind your ears.

You can move in gentle circles, stay in each area for a while, and eventually begin to make your way down the throat, following the sternocleidomastoid muscle that runs down your neck *(see image below)*.

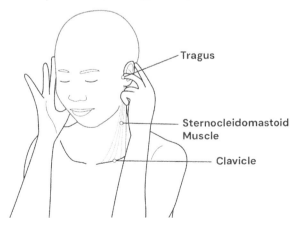

Tragus

Sternocleidomastoid Muscle

Clavicle

Take your time with the massage, and as you move down the neck muscle, move the ring finger away from the tragus and eventually use two fingers to massage this neck muscles with gentle circular movements. Move all the way down your neck until you get to your clavicles. Repeat this massage as many times as you like, as long as it feels comfortable. Always pay attention to how you feel before and after a practice. Journal if you have a bit of time or have any insights you would like to capture.

It's important to note that the activation of the vagus nerve and stimulation of a parasympathetic response, such as feeling more relaxed and calm, may happen after the first practice, or it may not happen immediately. Also, since we are all very different, what may work well for one may not work at all for another. You are absolutely invited to find and then stick with those methods that work best for you, and where you can find the quickest relief. There is no point in working with a practice that consistently has no effect on you. With this specific exercise, you may also find that the massage of different parts of the neck, or especially the massage behind the ears, works best for you. Stick with what works for you.

4. Neck Massage With the Help of a Ball

Instead of using your hands and fingers, the neck massage is often explained using a coregeous ball. For those that may not know, this is an inflatable air-filled sponge massage therapy ball that is great for massaging different parts of the body. If you don't have such a ball, you can use tennis balls, or another ball no bigger than the size of your neck. To perform the massage, slightly tilt your head to one side and place the ball on the side of the neck you are working on, just below your ear. Spin the ball slowly so it can gently massage and capture the soft tissue that lines the front of your neck. Go all the way across to the other side.

You are moving from just below one ear to just below the other, and are crossing that midline. Lighten your pressure around the midline, especially if you find the bones and tissue there more sensitive. Increase the pressure again once you are moving over the deeper muscle layer. Of course, you will need to slightly move your head as you are moving the ball, opening up the part of the neck that you are massaging. With this massage of the deeper tissue, you are ideally reaching a number of deeper underlying muscles that get heavily activated and generally overused in stress responses.

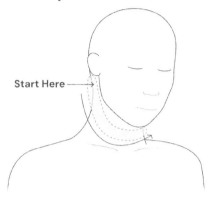

Do this massage for a couple of minutes and then feel into the body, specifically your neck. You may feel a sense of warmth or even tingling in the area around the neck. Also, take note of how this message affects you and how it feels on your face. For some people, this may even have a positive effect on their eyesight and hearing. Why not simply give this a try now? This may even become a go-to practice in the future, especially if you are a fan of massages and physical exercises for the body

5. Activation Through Pressure on the Clavicle

We will continue to move down the body now, working with the area around and just underneath the clavicle. It's best to do this practice standing. Move your arms and legs to loosen the body, and come up and down on your toes a few times. Move your head from side to side to help release any tension from it and neck. Stretch and then relax your shoulders by bringing them up and then back down. For this practice, you are going to be alternating between the right and left sides of the body.

Begin by placing your right hand just underneath your left clavicle. Place the flat of your hand on your skin and gently press down. Then carefully tilt your head to the right until you feel the stretch on the left side of the neck. You are again stretching the sternocleidomastoid muscle, which will help activate the vagus nerve. Hold this position for about 5–10 seconds, or a bit longer if you feel comfortable. Now switch sides, placing the left hand just underneath the right clavicle, and again applying a medium downward pressure. Tilt your head to the left this time and feel the stretch on the right side of your neck. If you don't really feel the stretch in your neck, apply a bit more downward pressure with your left hand or increase the tilt of your head. Practice on each side, roughly 5–10 sides. Do ensure that you practice an equal amount on both sides.

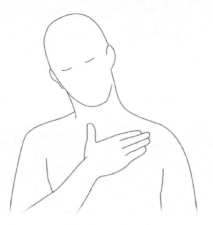

If you have ever been to a yoga class where these kinds of head and neck stretches are done at the beginning, and you remember feeling all relaxed and rejuvenated after only the first few minutes, now you know why. You were activating your vagus nerve, and therefore your parasympathetic nervous system. Through these simple stretches, your brain and body began sending signals back and forth that it is safe, and that it can relax! Yes, relaxation and calm can really be this simple, especially if you can do these practices with your eyes closed and can mostly turn off the active mind of thoughts and memories. If, of course, the mind presents you with troubling and difficult thoughts or even painful memories, things get a bit more tricky than this. I will address this more in depth in the chapters sharing practices and tools for working with trauma.

6. Butterfly Hug

Here is a simple, yet beautiful grounding technique that can support you in emotional times. Lift your hands in front of your chest and make sure your palms are facing you. The fingers are spread and you can wiggle them around a bit. Then have both thumbs gently touch, interlocking one behind the other. Your hands now resemble the wings of a butterfly, with your right hand now being in front of the left side of your chest and your left hand being in front of the right side of your chest. Then place both of your hands on your chest and begin alternating a gentle tap with one hand and then with the other. Take a look at the following image to see if you are doing it correctly.

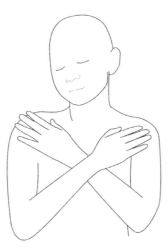

If you prefer, you can also place your hands on your upper arms. If this also does not feel comfortable, you can opt for placing your hands on your thighs and tap there. Before you begin, take a deep breath in through the nose, fill yourself up with fresh air, and then take a deep exhale, releasing any tension. Now begin with the practice. You can start to tap very slowly and gently, going at your own speed. Keep going for as long as it feels comfortable, varying tapping speed and strength a bit as feels natural.

I once did this practice with a 6'1" football player who would regularly have his anger get the better of him in our sessions. When I first told him what we were doing, he looked at me with irritation and disapproval and said, "I am not doing the butterfly hug." I challenged him a bit, knowing I might be able to get through to him with a little game. I told him that if he tried the practice and didn't like it or found it effective, he would never again have to try any of my sillier girly methods (as he called many of them). Having been drilled by his parents, boarding school and the military into being a tough man, he really struggled with being with and feeling his own emotions.

So what do you think happened? Well, the first time we did the practice, nothing did. As it often happens, he got quite angry in the session as he was remembering painful events from his childhood and how his girlfriend was triggering these emotions. I suggested he try the butterfly hug, and after a few minutes he preferred to stop, saying this wasn't working for him. I was a bit surprised and was wondering what I would do with him in the future, knowing that I could no longer use many of my more creative, "girly" methods.

When he came back the following week, he stormed into my office and said that I wouldn't believe what happened to him in the past week. It turned out that after our session, when he got home, he started to feel this immense sadness in his entire being. He said it was so strong, that there was nothing he could do to stop it, and then he just began crying. He said it wasn't even a specific memory and he didn't even really know what he was sad about, but that he'd never had such an experience in his life before. He mentioned he used the butterfly hug a few more times during the week when he got angry and upset, and found it to be working right away. He didn't have any more intense emotional moments like after the first time, but he was so baffled by how things developed after our last session that he just decided to continue doing the butterfly hug.

7. Butterfly Hug Using Affirmations

If you don't believe that the butterfly hug can work for you, I invite you to try this technique the next time you are finding yourself emotional. You can also try this method when you don't feel much at all or are lacking a sense of connection with yourself. If you remember the different vagus nerve pathways and which parts of the body they run through, you might remember that the ventral vagal pathway mainly runs through the face, throat and heart. Now what do you suppose happens when you continuously tap an area of your body that is associated with the ventral vagal pathway? Yes, exactly! The ventral vagal pathway gets activated through the tapping of the chest.

The butterfly hug also works because it is a form of bilateral stimulation of the brain. It activates and balances the activity between both sides of the brain. This technique is also a recommended practice in EMDR therapy, which can help access and process subconscious memories and associated emotions through the bilateral stimulation of the brain. Even Prince Harry has shared about using this technique in his therapy sessions.[11]

Another very beautiful add-on to this practice is attaching positive affirmations to the alternating tapping. Positive affirmations are positively loaded phrases that can help challenge unhelpful or negative thoughts. So you could be doing the gentle tapping while you say, for example, "I am safe" or "I am loved." This may feel a bit odd or even fake at first, so keep going through the awkward phase. Then, after some time, check in with yourself to see how you are feeling and if you would like to continue.

Positive affirmations work for some people, but not for others. So even though there might be some initial resistance to begin with, after a time the amount of resistance should decrease. Speaking out loud affirmations that your brain is really resisting, even after some time, might actually be counterproductive. So give it a try and see how using the butterfly hug and positive affirmations works for you. Maybe only one of the two really resonates, and that is okay.

8. The Pillow Hug

Have you ever felt sad or lonely and found yourself looking for comfort by hugging something like a stuffed animal or a pillow? When someone else hugs us, this generally reduces our cortisol levels (our stress hormone) and helps release oxytocin. But what can we do when no one is available? Or even if people are, and we simply do not feel safe or comforted by the idea of hugging them? Believe it or not, hugging an object or a pillow can have similar and comforting effects.[12] Also, how many of us actually hug a pillow at night, especially when we are separated from our romantic partners?

It is likely that a similar automatic, unconscious self-soothing attempt is the reason for this. Obviously, this won't work with everyone, especially while having sessions. People really need to feel safe and ready for what some consider more of a child-like practice. Yet, children choose these practices for a reason. Their smart little bodies do all the things they need to in order to feel safe and protected, no matter how silly it may look.

Why not try this now for just a few moments? If you feel this practice is silly or "too easy," you can make this "more difficult" by thinking of something that recently upset you or something you are still angry about before the practice. Imagine this situation, the people involved, and then seek comfort and support by hugging a pillow. Make sure you work with a situation of light to medium emotional charge only, especially when doing this for the first time. Think of the situation (if you are working with one) and then hug the pillow or a stuffed animal and press it tightly against your chest. How does the pillow or stuffed animal feel when pressed against your body? Remove the object for a moment and notice the difference. If you are working with a situation, remind yourself of the situation while hugging the pillow or stuffed animal and, if you feel ready, try it again when not hugging any object. Do you notice any differences?

If you put aside any sense of feeling silly or childish, how does it really make you feel? It's probably quite comforting. Too bad that as adults we are often more focused on what other people think, instead of taking care of our wellbeing. Just imagine what would happen if people started taking their comforting pillow into the office. I believe it could be a very insightful and effective experiment.

9. Hand Over Your Heart

Similarly to the last practice of hugging a pillow or a stuffed animal, a self-soothing touch such as placing a hand over your heart works in a very similar way.[13] For thousands of years, placing your hand over your heart has been a symbol of honesty and sincerity. We make such a gesture when we are touched emotionally, both positively and also negatively. Often it is also a sign of personal dismay.

I would like to include some simple practices in accordance with this that are also known to bring about a deeper connection with ourselves.

- Simply place one or both hands over your heart. For example, you can simply place your right hand over your heart while keeping your hand flat. There is no need to apply any kind of pressure; simply placing the hand here for around 5–10 seconds can help us to feel within and connect with ourselves. Self-connection means being aware of how we feel inside, and accepting the status quo of these feelings. So use this practice as a form of self-connection. It may feel a bit weird at first, but just give it a try. If you use both hands, it's best to keep the right hand on the bottom and the left hand on top.

- Do Anjali Mudra or the so-called prayer pose, as these are practiced in yoga. This has nothing to do with actually praying, but is simply a form of recognition of ourselves and of others. You simply bring your palms together in front of your chest. The fingers are touching and are slightly spread apart. You can apply a little bit of pressure with your thumbs to your sternum. Open the chest by bringing the shoulders up and back, and breathe deeply in and out. Close your eyes if possible and remain in this posture for 3–6 minutes.

- During either practice, pay attention to the sensations that arise in the chest area. Feel the connection to your heart and see if anything else arises.

Now finish both or either practice and journal how you feel.

10. Activation of the Body

The first ten tools of this chapter on supporting self-regulation through touch focused, for the most part, on the vagus nerve stimulation that will help you calm and relax. They supported the down regulation of the nervous system from sympathetic to parasympathetic activation. So many of the previous practices can be used when you are finding yourself upset, angry or in any way emotional that does not feel supportive at the moment.

Now what if you find yourself stuck in immobility or a freeze response? Take this example of a former client of mine. Deborah had had a severe car accident when she was in her 20s. Almost 20 years later, she regularly has moments while driving that remind her of the accident where she completely freezes up. She will pass a specific landmark or a certain type of car coming from the other direction, and the dorsal vagal shutdown will activate. Now you can imagine that while driving, this can be not only dangerous but actually life-threatening to her and others around her. For Deborah, these moments of freeze are only micro moments, of just a few milliseconds. The moment she becomes aware of her freeze reaction, she will help herself out of it. Being able to do this doesn't happen overnight, of course.

The following three tools will focus on the up regulation of the nervous system. From dorsal vagal shutdown back to parasympathetic rest and digest. If you remember the ladder, you will remember that people need to move through all three steps or stages. The following are just a few tools to help bring quick relief. In chapters 3 and 4 when I address working with trauma, I will give much more detail on this.

So what's the first thing that you can do when you notice yourself going into a freeze-or-collapse response? Well, first of all, it's good that you are aware. No matter if it's a mean comment from your boss or your long-term partner making weekend plans with his friends without telling you, if something someone else does causes you to freeze or collapse, you know that there is something here for you to learn. Something is being triggered; something is being activated. Even though it may seem really uncomfortable, you might rather want to escape that situation at that moment. I understand and often still feel the same.

Now, one very simple thing that you can do as you find yourself going into the freeze/collapse response is to actually initiate a slight activation of the body. Just simply begin to move your arms and legs a little, or see if you can get up and just take a few steps. If none of this is available, see if you can gently move your head from side to side. Any kind of movement will do, really. Please make sure not to make any abrupt movements. You are trying to move from freezing into rest and calm. Abrupt movements and/or screaming, for example, are likely to have you moving into sympathetic activation. This can also have its purpose, and we will speak more about this later.

11. Reconnecting Body with the Floor

For most people, a freeze or collapse response often comes with a form of dissociation from the body and mind. You are simply not connected to yourself or to the world around you. I will address these topics and ideas in detail when we speak about trauma. Whether you feel you have experienced traumatic events or not, many of us have this tendency to "check out" regularly for a few moments. Technically, there is nothing wrong with this, it's just that most people are happiest when they feel connected to themselves and the present. In sessions, clients will often share, when speaking about difficult or traumatic memories, that it literally felt like someone pulled the rug from underneath them. This is what this freeze-or-collapse response can feel like, if it feels like anything at all.

What can you do in those moments where you feel like you have lost touch with a solid surface to stand on? Well, the simplest way is to try to re-establish the connection with this place of support. Using imagination and the sense of touch, you try to reestablish a solid place to stand. We can even try this together, whether you feel grounded or not. Such a practice is known to give energy and generally activate the body. Read the instructions below or for a more seamless experience I've gone ahead and created a guided audio for this exercise.

You can access it by scanning the following QR code or using this url: *https://bit.ly/ptmadesimple*

- Find yourself a chair or somewhere to sit. Ideally, you can do this practice somewhere you feel comfortable and safe, and where you don't have to worry about others watching or looking at you.

- Start by sitting up straight and doing little movements with the head, neck and torso to warm up. Then place your hands on your thighs and simply begin feeling your feet. Just feel the outline of both of your feet.

- Then begin to focus on the right foot and, following the outline of it, start to let your attention move around your right foot. See where it touches the ground. Investigate for yourself where most of the weight of the right foot is resting. Are you mainly standing on your heel or on your toes, or is the weight evenly distributed?

- Do the exact same thing with your left foot. Follow the outline of it and begin to let your attention move around it. See where your left foot touches the ground. Investigate for yourself where most of the weight of the left foot is resting. Are you mainly standing on your heel or on your toes, or is the weight evenly distributed?

- Now gently move your feet a little and come up on your toes a few times. Check in on how your feet and body feel.

- Next, you are going to ground yourself through both feet, really focusing on their connection with the ground underneath them. See how the ground feels and if it can evenly support the weight of the body. You can even imagine that there are roots growing out of your feet, connecting you with the ground. Feel the sense of stability and strength this practice brings. Keep on making the connection with the ground, close your eyes if you can, and just feel this sense of grounding and support.

- Doing something like you just did can be extremely supportive to calm and also get fresh energy into the system. Now, as a last part of this practice to help the activation of the nervous system, lift one leg after another, raising one, letting it fall down, and then raising the other. Just gently lift and drop your legs. Do this practice on each leg five times. You are likely to notice a stronger activation in the body as a result, as well as a sense of connection and grounding. It will be very hard to remain dissociated and cut off if you can do this practice.

12. Barefoot Walk in Nature

When was the last time you walked barefoot outside? A little stroll through your garden or even over to your neighbor's house? Have you ever actually left your house without shoes? If you ever have the chance to spend a bit more time in tropical countries or some spiritual communities, you will find a lot of people walking barefooted. Some people stop wearing shoes completely. I remember a man in my hometown who would never wear shoes, no matter if it was the middle of the summer or during the snowy winters. Walking barefoot enhances your proprioception, or your ability to perceive your body in space. It is great for balance and overall posture, and should you ever try it, you will notice it is also great for the soul. Especially when walking over soft surfaces, like freshly mowed grass or mildly warm sand. And walking over such surfaces doesn't only feel good, it also activates the vagus nerve, helping you calm down and relax.

From a yogic perspective, the direct contact with the ground provides a sense of support and stability, easing anxiety and stress.

So here is the invitation: Take a 10–15-minute barefoot walk outdoors. You can go to your favorite park in shoes if you prefer, and simply take them off when you get there. Now you can just walk over the grass. Or, if your feet are not so sensitive, you can simply leave the house without shoes and go around a couple of blocks. You can also go into the forest if the ground is not too prickly or covered in sharp rocks. Make sure you do this during a time of the day and year when it is not too cold outside.

Start with softer surfaces and then work your way to harder ones as you have more practice. Start with only 5–7 minutes if your feet are very sensitive, and work your way toward longer walks over time. If you have the opportunity, next time it rains and is not too cold, go outside in your yard or a nearby garden to walk in the rain, specifically through the grass. This can be very beautiful and is also very playful. If it rains a lot, and you have the opportunity to step into bigger puddles, especially mud-puddles, even better. Kids know why they love to step and play in these. It's not only fun, but also soothing for the nervous system. Just take good care not to step into any sharp object and thoroughly wash your feet after.

During the walk, ask yourself the following questions:

1. What does it feel like when my feet are touching this surface?
    Come to stand for a moment and really feel into the ground and reflect.

2. What other surfaces can I try to step on?

3. How can I make this more playful?

Here you are activating the body by walking, which can help you out of a freeze or collapse response. Plus the connection with the ground, specifically the soft and comforting surfaces, help you relax and send signals to the body that you are safe.

13. Activation Through Tapping

Let me share with you one more short practice in this chapter that is almost guaranteed to get your energy up and help you move out of any kind of freeze or collapse response. Do this practice while standing up. You are simply going to take a deep breath in through the belly and then up into the chest. Hold your breath at the top, create some tension in the rib cage, and then use your fingers and wrists to begin tapping all over your upper body, specifically your chest, the sides and where you can reach on your back. During the tapping, keep holding your breath in.

When you can't hold your breath anymore, exhale deeply. Then immediately go into a new round, starting with a deep inhale through the belly. You can choose the speed and strength of the tapping, but obviously, the faster and harder you tap (without creating any pain, of course), the stronger the activation of the sympathetic nervous system. You can even ask someone, like your partner or child, to help you with this practice. This can also make some great laughs together.

What's interesting is that you can increase your threshold for being in a sympathetic state with this practice. We will explore other, more systematic forms of tapping later in the workbook.

PART 3

Polyvagal Theory to Work With Trauma

In these first chapters, you discovered the basics about PVT and nervous system regulation and dysregulation, respectively. I shared and invited you to try out a series of tools supporting self-regulation through your breath and self-touch. These next few chapters will focus on further applying PVT to working with and overcoming trauma. Bessel van der Kolk, M.D., describes trauma as the enduring imprint of past pain, horror, and fear rather than merely a historical event. According to the CDC, a significant portion of Americans have faced childhood sexual abuse, physical violence leaving marks, or domestic violence at some point.

Many children grow up in environments marked by alcohol abuse or witness domestic violence, which can profoundly impact their development.[14] Today, we understand that trauma extends beyond experiences like war or severe physical violence, and the individual reactions and long-term consequences of experienced trauma differ as much as individuals do. Whatever made you pick up this book and find out how PVT can potentially help you or your clients, know that you are not alone when it comes to having gone through and being impacted by trauma.

Let's take a closer look to understand how PVT can be used to explain trauma reactions and trauma recovery. Imagine the following scenario: Jenny is now in her late 20s and grew up with both of her parents. Their relationship was characterized by constant ups and downs, shouting fights and frequent shifts between loving and hating each other. When Jenny came home from school, she never knew what the situation would be like. One day they would be one big happy family, joyfully sharing and laughing at the dinner table; the next would be characterized by dead silence, resentment and disapproval.

The way her parents were relating directly to each other would usually carry over to their interactions with their children. Ideally, a home is a place where we can relax and know that we are safe. For Jenny, coming home was full of uncertainties and unknowns. She didn't know whether she would be greeted or ignored by her mother, or be walking into a shouting match. She didn't know whether her father would show interest in her that day or project the anger he had for her mother onto Jenny.

Early on, Jenny's nervous system learned to be constantly on guard when in the "safety" of her own home. Looking at this from the lens of the nervous system and the nervous system's reaction, Jenny's nervous system learned early on that it needed to be alert and ready to fight or flee at all times. At school, Jenny would often just fall asleep in class or pick fights with her classmates, even teachers. You could say that her sympathetic nervous system was overly active. Jenny had no real safe space or a place where she could relax, so over time the relaxed parasympathetic response would get less and less, and the switch between parasympathetic and sympathetic responses was simply not working anymore.

Wherever Jenny would go, she would feel tense and anxious, ready to protect herself when needed. After many years of constant tension and stress, she started to develop back pain and recurring migraines. Episodes of pain would suddenly occur without any warning and often diffusely affect her entire body. Her sympathetic response was maxed out as the parasympathetic dorsal shut-down response was activated. The body couldn't sustain the constant release of stress hormones, bodily tension and worrying thoughts. Over the years, Jenny's body simply became sick, and her sympathetic nervous system would react and take over in almost all areas of life. Being in a state of tension and anxiety felt so normal for her that she even unconsciously brought this into different situations in her life, specifically relationships.

Whether you are struggling with trauma related to ongoing or one-time experiences, PVT suggests that we need to come back into the appropriate nervous system response. For this to happen, generally, the cascade of and relationship between ventral vagal parasympathetic response, sympathetic response and dorsal vagal parasympathetic shut-down needs to be clearly seen and, in many cases, re-experienced. To come back into the ventral vagal relaxed parasympathetic response, we often need to come back up the ladder and move from dorsal vagal shutdown to sympathetic response, and eventually into a reaction of safety and calm connected to the ventral vagal pathways of the parasympathetic nervous system. The purpose of these next two chapters is to present you with a series of tools that can support you exactly in this. For a simplified overview and understanding, we will separate tools into one chapter focusing on tools to help you out of the dorsal vagal shut-down and another on sharing tools on how to move through the sympathetic activation back into ventral vagal social engagement.

CHAPTER 3

Coming Out of Dorsal Shut-Down

When someone experiences trauma, this often interrupts the autonomic nervous system's regulation. In many cases, people become hypersensitive in their reactions and, for example, begin perceiving threats where there are none. So even a safe environment, such as a lively café you visit with your friends, with lots of chatter and laughter, could feel dangerous and potentially threatening. After reading the first few chapters, you know that PVT works at the level of the physical body. While we will continue this body-based healing approach in the tools presented over the next chapters, let's begin this first chapter on PVT tools for trauma recovery, specifically movement out of the dorsal shut-down, with gaining a better understanding of your trauma reactions and bodily responses.

1. Tapping Into the Body and Bodily Cues

When we feel as though our minds, emotions or bodies have simply been taken over and reactions are outside of our control, it is likely that something challenging or even traumatic from the past is at play. Our actions and reactions seem to be fully out of our conscious awareness, especially when the nervous system has initiated the dorsal vagal shut-down. For this reason, you need to better understand your personal responses to actual and perceived stressors and threats. Let's explore this a bit more in the next practice of tracking your own body cues. You can do the following exercise any time. The more you do such a practice, the easier you will find these little check-ins of the body.

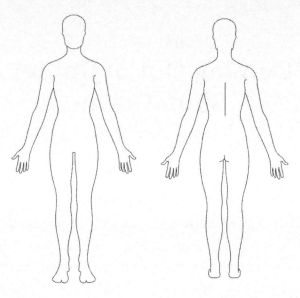

Areas of Discomfort   **Areas of Activation**

_____

_____

_____

_____

_____

_____

_____

1. Looking at the image above, mark any areas of discomfort, pain or numbness in the body using one color.

2. Then mark any areas of activation, tingling, buzzing or feeling warm in another color.

3. Write down the specific areas of the body where perceptions are strongest and note down exactly what you are feeling.

As you first begin doing such a practice it might seem tricky. You are likely not to feel much of anything at all, especially if you are in dorsal vagal shutdown. But remember that even feeling a sense of numbness in the body means you are perceiving something. The purpose of doing such a practice is to invite you into reconnection with and feeling of the body. If we did not learn this at an early age, as is the case for many adults, we will have to go back and learn to first sense and eventually interpret the cues of the body. Please take good care if you should find yourself overwhelmed by the type and amount of sensations you are experiencing while doing this exercise. Should this be the case, move onto practice number 5, which will help you back into safety and orientation.

2. Is My Nervous System Dysregulated?

Now let's continue exploring your body and tracking any cues, specifically when finding yourself in dorsal vagal shut-down. You may ask whether you are finding yourself in this state often characterized by signs of freeze, numbness, maybe even dissociation. How can you even tell? Very good question, and to begin, you may not be able to. Many people may not even know that their nervous system is dysregulated, and that this may actually be the cause for why they are experiencing little energy and motivation, even lethargy and a sense of disconnection from others.

I have worked with many clients who thought they had absolutely no problems or difficulties in life, despite having experienced one-time or chronic trauma, because they were simply feeling nothing—nothing at all. It was as if they were cut off from their bodies, and felt sensations and emotions other than through mental explanation. Over the course of time and working together this shifted, and clients started perceiving sensations and emotions very differently. This turnabout came with its fair amount of challenges to start, of course.

As a first step, it is good for you to understand whether your nervous system is actually regulated or dysregulated at a given instance. As mentioned, you may think you are doing fine, feeling calm and relaxed, yet when you look closer or begin to check in more frequently, it is not so.

There are countless signs of potential nervous system dysregulation; let's take a look at a few. Please read the statements below and mark for yourself or together with your client which of the statements are "true."

- You feel like you are often experiencing an emotional rollercoaster of very strong emotions and extreme mood swings, and have a hard time controlling your emotions. _____

- You find yourself often overreacting to certain situations, or you find yourself hypersensitive to certain stimuli. _____

- You have a hard time sleeping (falling or staying asleep). _____

- You have a hard time controlling your impulses or making decisions. _____

- You have physical symptoms such as feeling tired, irritable, tense or even in pain. _____

Of course, I could add many more questions to this list, but these questions focus on core aspects of nervous system regulation, such as emotional reaction, impulsivity, physical symptoms, sleep problems and reactivity.

Remember that a dysregulated nervous system is one that is in a state of activation that is not in alignment with the needs of the current situation. When we are walking through a dark alley at night and are feeling anxious and tense, this can be seen as a very adequate response of the nervous system, as the sympathetic activation will have us ready for fight or flight at any point. If we are feeling the same anxiety and tension when we are in a room full of puppies, something is likely to be up.

3. Sympathetic or Parasympathetic Activation

One of the first things I like to explore with clients is to help them better understand their bodies and the signs their bodies are sending them. On countless occasions, I would ask clients how they were feeling and what they were perceiving in the body, and I often received responses such as, "Oh, I am feeling pretty good" or "I don't feel much of anything right now." Just observing these clients and feeling a bit of the energy shift as they entered the room, I could often see clear signs of stress and tension, such as a clenching of the jaw or fist or seeing clients fidget in their chairs.

It takes some years of practice, but after working with hundreds of clients on the most common health conditions and struggles, at some point you know when the spoken word does not match what is being perceived and felt. Many of us can feel this in others without any kind of training. We can clearly feel it in our best friends or someone close to us when they tell us they are fine but actually have something on their chests. The same kind of sensitivity and perception need to be brought into our own bodies to observe and interpret bodily signs.

Take a look at the following graphic and see which of these signs or symptoms are true for you at this moment. You can mark each aspect with a colored pen and then see how many aspects suggest parasympathetic activation and how many may relate to sympathetic activation.

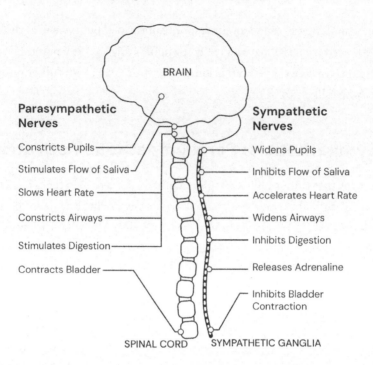

Would you say that your sympathetic or parasympathetic nervous system is active right now?

_____

_____

Why?

_____

_____

4. Simple Questions for a Body Check-In

I know some of these practices can be difficult, even frustrating, to start. If the sensitivity and practice is not there, you might be feeling very little or the same kind of bodily symptoms every time. Yet with practice, you will notice that the perception of the body and its symptoms becomes more fine-tuned and you are able to perceive more nuances of bodily symptoms, even emotions. Remember that if you or a client have experienced trauma in the past that your system could not handle at the time, then it was your nervous system that likely initiated a shut-down response with the intention of ensuring your survival.

As you continue this journey into better understanding your bodily responses and nervous system regulation, here are a few questions that can support you in this. If you like, you can ask yourself the questions right now and then journal your responses. For the future, you can simply do these reflection questions at any place and time randomly, mentally answering yourself.

1. Take a moment to let your attention move through your entire body. You can move from down up and from up down. What do you notice? Does your attention rest anywhere specifically?

_____

_____

_____

_____

2. Continue bringing your attention inward, scanning the different body parts. What parts of your body feel light and open?

_____

_____

_____

_____

3. What parts of your body feel closed and contracted?

_____

_____

_____

_____

4. Where (if) do you feel any tension?

_____

_____

_____

_____

5. What else do you notice or perceive?

_____

_____

_____

_____

6. How is the quality of your mind?

_____

_____

_____

_____

5. Coming Back into Presence

When doing these kinds of practices and connecting with and feeling into the body we may go from not feeling at all, to suddenly feeling a lot, even being overwhelmed by what we experience. As it is important to gradually move back up the ladder into sympathetic activation and not overwhelm the nervous system even more than it already has been, we need practices helping us to come back into safety through connecting with the present moment. You can do the following practice at any point in time if you are feeling overwhelmed by what you are experiencing, perceiving or remembering. This also works great when working with clients, when you notice that they go into a state of sympathetic overactivation or are dissociating. It's really simple, yet extremely effective.

You are simply invited to look around the room and answer the following for yourself, or have your clients answer:

- Name something you find beautiful in this room.

- Name something with the color green.

- Notice the color and shape of your chair.

- Name something that you would like to inspect further.

If you find yourself getting caught up in certain memories, thoughts, sensations or emotions, you may find that even answering only one or two of these will help you calm down and bring you back into the present moment.

6. Activate the Senses

Dorsal vagal shut-down can be a temporary, short term state in an acute situation, or it can also become a chronic condition. Of course, it is generally easier to come out of a temporary short term shut-down compared to having lived in such a state for many years. When beginning to uncover underlying topics, triggers or wounds with clients or patients, clients may temporarily slip into dorsal vagal shut-down. Sometimes it's hard to tell if they weren't already in a state of shut-down before, and now just entered a deeper form that is characterized by more obvious symptoms of numbness, disconnection and even dissociation. In my first years of supporting clients, these kinds of moments would sometimes overwhelm me, as I could feel that my clients had completely checked out and I wasn't sure how to bring them back. Maybe their physical bodies were still in the room, sitting on the chair across from me, but the person was no longer mentally or emotionally present.

Here is a story from my client Anne that illustrates such a scenario very well. Please note that the following recount may be triggering for some people. If you don't feel like you are in a good space at the moment, feeling grounded and stable, just skip the next page. I had been speaking to Anne about her difficult relationship with her father for a few sessions and she always amazed me with how reflected she was. She would recall exactly how she felt and what she would have needed instead. It seemed as though she had it all figured out, and yet I had a feeling that something was there that was causing her to have current relationships with men that were characterized by mistrust and disbelief.

As she was recalling the events of one summer holiday with her father, she started remembering a situation at a campground. In the middle of her story, Anne suddenly froze up, and her face became blank. It was as if someone had taken all her thoughts and ideas and simply put her on pause. I called her name a few times to bring her back to the present moment, which more or less worked. I often recommend this simple measure to partners or spouses of persons suffering from trauma, PTSD, C-PTSD or dissociative disorders. Anne tried to continue with her story but simply lost her thoughts, not remembering well what she wanted to share next. It was the first week of January, and I had brought lots of left-over chocolate and cookies from the Christmas holidays back to the office. Suddenly, I had the inspiration to offer Anne one of the cookies.

We put talking about the memory aside and just remained in the present moment for some minutes, eating a few cookies and refreshing ourselves with cool water. After a few moments, Anne continued her story without me asking. "We were at our favorite campground in the mountains and had just packed all of our camping gear, ready to leave and drive back home," she said. "We were already in the car driving away when I realized I urgently needed to go to the bathroom. When I went to check, I found the women's restroom closed due to cleaning, and the cleaning lady telling me to go to the men's restroom right next door. I didn't want to go there by myself, so I asked my father to come with me and wait outside the bathroom stall. He said I would be fine and sent me off by myself. I remember asking again, really wanting him to come with me, but he just made a humorous response and told me to hurry up. So I went by myself.

When I went inside, I felt fearful and anxious, and right as I was entering the bathroom, I saw a man urinate right in front of me. He just winked at me, then continued on with his business. I went to the bathroom, absolutely terrified. I had just seen the genitals of a man that I don't even know, all because my father wouldn't come with me to the bathroom. He is supposed to protect me, but he is the one who sent me into this situation alone. Not all of these insights came at exactly this moment, of course, but years later, this specific memory haunted me again and again in my dreams. I never told my father what happened, but my trust in him (and men in general from then on) had been broken."

Here is what happened from my perspective: Anne had really recalled this memory in our session. At this time, we are not just mentally recalling what happened but actually re-experiencing the sensations and emotions that were associated with this memory. The moment the body realized the intensity of what was happening, Anne's nervous system initiated a shut-down response to protect her from the overwhelm she had likely also felt when she was 8 years old and needed to enter the men's bathroom all by herself and saw a stranger urinate in front of her. Instead of focusing on finding out more and interrogating her about what she was experiencing and remembering, I offered her some cookies and a glass of water.

Anne was able to come back to the present moment and remember that she was safe and that she was no longer an 8-year-old little girl. After she finished her cookie, she continued the story fully on her own, without my guidance or asking. Her body and her nervous system were ready to recall and re-experience the traumatic events.

This might be a long story to share with you a very simple tool, yet it was a pivotal point in my work with clients, as it allowed me to support them back into the present moment, while ensuring that they were able to move through a situation in their own time. It helped me see the importance of guiding clients back into safety first, before they can re-experience or process any difficult or especially traumatic memory.

If you are reading this and are not working with clients, this practice can still be very helpful for you. Say you are noticing that you suddenly feel numb or disconnected, this is how you can help yourself back into the present moment in the exact same way by activating the senses. Whether perhaps you have a yummy treat or a refreshing glass of lemon water, smell your favorite perfume or flower, or simply run your hands through freshly cut grass is up to you. The intention is to activate your senses and bring you back into the here and now.

7. Accept and Embrace the Shut-Down

If you read and tried out the last practice, you may have understood a very important element of helping yourself or your clients come out of dorsal vagal shut-down. Do you know what it could be? I mean the importance of accepting and embracing the current condition of the body. Remember that the body is simply trying to protect you and ensure your survival. In moments like the one I was recalling about Anne in the last practice, her body simply initiated a shut-down response at the moment she really went back into the memory and began feeling the associated emotions.

While in this story it was not really an active form of acceptance we were practicing, I was encouraging the reconnection with her adult self, making her feel safe enough to share further memories of her own. What can it look like when you are actively accepting and embracing a dorsal vagal shutdown? I will try to guide you through this in this short practice. Please be aware that such a practice is likely to be easier when supported by a professional. The difficulty with a dorsal vagal shutdown is that people often struggle to identify such a state by themselves. Here is a step-by-step approach that I have shared with clients in the past when they were looking for guidance and support while at home and without my support.

Identify your dorsal vagal shut-down symptoms

Everyone's symptoms of a dorsal vagal shut-down are different. As you or your clients are on their healing path, it becomes critical to become more and more familiar, even intimate with the unique symptoms. At first, it might be hard to name and pinpoint these yourself, but as you start to pay more attention, ask others to support you or are working with a professional, you will be better able to name and observe the symptoms that indicate a dorsal shutdown for you.

Remember that symptoms can be in the form of thinking, sensations, emotions and impulses (things that you do). Some people feel numb or disconnected; others simply feel unmotivated. Some may feel heavy, while others may feel like they are floating. Some may not feel many emotions or sensations, but they may be heavily isolating themselves from their surroundings. For many, it's a combination or mix of all of these. Pay attention to the symptoms that you typically experience. Generally, you are able to recall these better just as you are about to come out of dorsal shut-down or as mentioned when working with a professional.

Identify if you have the capacity to help yourself out of dorsal vagal shut-down, or whether you need support

Once you have identified that you are finding yourself in a dorsal shut-down response, you need to answer one very important question: Do you currently have the capacity to hold space for and support yourself out of this state? Do you feel confident enough to handle this situation on your own, or do you need support? If you are not sure, as with most questions in life, "not sure" is not a "yes," so best assume it's a "no." You don't always need to work with a professional, and the last chapter of this workbook will entail many tools for how you can be helped by a compassionate and supportive friend or even partner.

Find yourself a safe space for the rest of the practice

You will need some moments of alone and quiet time for this practice. Ensure that you have a private space that will work for you. I can tell you that with time, you are likely to be able to do such practices in a public restroom or even in a public park. To begin, it's best to find a private space that you know and where you feel safe.

Fully accept and embrace the symptoms and the situation

Get comfortable in your safe space and find somewhere where you can sit or lie down. For some people, it may work better to very slowly walk in circles as they do the practice. Begin by taking a few deep breaths, and then place your right hand over your heart. Breathe a bit deeper and longer than you naturally would, so you can feel your hand rise and fall. Then begin saying to yourself the following words: "Even though I don't feel *good/comfortable/ happy/connected* right now, I fully accept and embrace the current situation. I fully accept and embrace feeling *numb, disconnected/alone/heavy/unmotivated/isolated/etc.*

Replace the words in italics with a word or words that best describe your situation. Keep repeating these two sentences for a few minutes. You can slightly adjust the wording or add sentences that spontaneously come to mind. Just ensure that they are really supporting you in accepting and embracing the situation. Note that this may work for you the first time you do it, or it may not work at all. There might be resistance coming up and symptoms that actually feel worse as you give them more space and direct attention. This is normal, and you will find that with time, you can move through such situations more easily. Still, use your discernment in deciding if you do need professional support at any point and time you feel overwhelmed.

Give yourself permission to move out of the dorsal vagal shut-down

Sometimes the body needs a bit of extra encouragement to signal that it's safe to move out of dorsal vagal shut-down. In some cases, the mind even seems to hold us in the shut-down response as a way of "protection." In many of these cases, the mind will say it's not possible or safe to come out of the shut-down. Coming out of a shut-down response and back into feeling emotions that are often associated with the sympathetic nervous system, or back into connecting socially with others, can also be scary.

So for some people, being and staying in dorsal vagal shut-down may have become an unconscious strategy or a form of self-sabotage. If this is the case, it will become necessary that you become aware of this and give yourself permission to move out of the shut-down response. This may take a bit of practice and may need to be supported by a professional. As a start, you can simply write down and repeat the following statement: "I fully give myself permission to move out of the shut-down response." Or, "I am ready to move out of the shut-down or freeze response."

Trust in the wisdom of the body and that everything happens at the right time

I stated this at the beginning of this workbook and will state it again here. It was the body's wisdom that protected you initially, and it will be the body's wisdom that will help you out of this again. Yes, perceptions and reactions of the body may still be quite off and need to be re-calibrated, but this is a process and will take time. Inviting a sense of trust in your own body and its wisdom is the best prerequisite for the body to allow itself to move through and process anything it may need to in order to come out of the dorsal shut-down. Of course, it's naive to think that the body will handle all of this on its own without any support, but re-establishing a loving and trusting relationship with their bodies has brought wonders to some of my clients, and even myself.

8. Finding Your Safety State

As I mentioned in the last few practices, in order to come out of dorsal vagal shut-down, it is important to accept how you are feeling and what you are experiencing. Just as important is re-creating a sense of safety and protection on the outside to suggest to the body that it can feel safe to move out of the shut-down. You may have your own ideas and ways to make yourself feel safe and protected; in case you do not, here is a list of things that you can refer to in moments when you find yourself frozen, collapsed or numb, and need help re-creating this sense of safety.

- **Wrap yourself in a cozy blanket.** The physical sensation of being wrapped up can provide a sense of security.

- **Hold a warm cup of tea.** The warmth and aroma can be soothing and comforting. Also, just the fact that we are holding something gives us something to do and invites us to come back to the present moment.

- **Pet an animal.** If you have a pet, spend time stroking or cuddling them. If you don't have any pets, see if there is a petting zoo nearby that you can go to.

- **Lie on the floor on your left side, gently bending your knees and hugging yourself.** This restorative yoga posture is commonly done at the end of a full-body relaxation. The self-hug in this position can feel extremely supportive and comforting.

- **Wear comfortable, snug clothing.** Clothes like a favorite hoodie or soft socks can make you feel safe and cozy.

- **Hug a tree.** Go outside and hug a tree. I know this might feel very strange, and you may only want to practice this before and after sunrise to begin so nobody sees you, but this really works. This is said to release Oxytocin, a comforting cuddle hormone, just as if we were hugging humans.[15]

- **Take a warm bath.** Allow your body to relax in the warm water, ideally using some relaxing and comforting smells. Ensure that you only do this if you feel safe in the water.

Please note that all of these suggestions do not include other people supporting you. Of course, for many of us, connecting with someone we love and trust is a hugely comforting and supportive factor. More on this in the last part on co-regulation.

9. Inviting a Light Muscle Tension

Safety, acceptance and embrace are critical to moving out of dorsal shut-down. Now what if you, like many who are specifically suffering from trauma, PTSD or C-PTSD, are not feeling anything at all? Maybe you just recently learned that your nervous system is dysregulated, and you have been spending most of your life in dorsal shut-down. If this is the case, please don't get discouraged.

Many of the practices that have previously been mentioned that activate the vagus nerve through the breath or touch are likely to work for you. Maybe not immediately, but over time, they will. Patience and persistence need to become your two new best friends. Stick with what feels good and celebrate even the tiniest little moments of success. Also, be aware that the journey may take some time, and you may need support from a professional. It is likely to take time to be fully healed and integrated, especially if you have experienced trauma over a longer period of time, and you may find yourself still having some limitations in everyday life even after years of healing.

If you do not feel yourself, if you feel numb or disconnected, and if you maybe don't even feel like you are in your body, I will share with you the following three very simple practices that all have a similar intention: to use conscious movement to help you come out of a freeze response. Remember that in a freeze response, your brain is in survival mode. Higher cognitive functioning is turned off, so you can't just tell yourself to get out of the freeze response. Since your body is causing you to stay in the freeze response, you need to signal your body that it is safe to move out of the dorsal vagal shut-down. The best way to do this is to communicate directly with the body through light movement.

- First, you can do this by simply tensing up different parts of your body. You can start by simply tensing up your hand. Just clench your right fist for a moment.

- Then continue with the left fist. Clench both fists, and then include the arms.

- Continue with tensing your toes, then feet and then legs.

- Tense your belly, then tense your buttocks.

- See what other areas of your body you can tense up.

- Take a moment to feel into anything that may arise after this practice.

1. How does the body feel after such a practice?

_____

_____

_____

_____

2. What thoughts, emotions or sensations arose during this practice?

_____

_____

_____

_____

10. Gentle Stretching

In dorsal vagal shut-down, your body is literally stuck or frozen in the belief that it is not safe to move, as any kind of movement could mean life-threatening danger. Interestingly, this is an evolutionary response that not only humans show. Guinea pigs and rabbits, as well as a number of snakes, actually play dead when they are captured by their predators. The moment their predator is not attentive, they quickly come back to life and attempt their escape. Similarly, the human shut-down or freeze response is an evolutionary adaptation. For the body, it is not safe to continue with its normal functioning.

The sympathetic fight-or-flight response can no longer guarantee a person's survival, as cortisol release and the experienced symptoms simply get too much for the system. The only option is a full shut-down. The solution: movement, movement, movement. This is being emphasized here as it is such a critical part of the polyvagal theory and part of the somatic therapy using PVT. In this practice, you are encouraged to stretch your body.

And by stretching the body, I mean stretching the entire body. This can easily take 15 minutes and should be done daily, no matter if you are in dorsal vagal shutdown or not. It keeps the body young and healthy.

Here is a simple stretching routine that you can follow. Read the instructions below or alternatively you can listen to the guided audio for this exercise accessibly scanning the following QR code or by using this url: *https://bit.ly/ptmadesimple*

Please adjust any of the stretches to your specific needs and fitness level.

1. **Neck Stretch:** Gently tilt your head to the right, bringing your ear toward your shoulder. Hold for 5-10 seconds, then repeat on the left side.

2. **Shoulder Rolls:** Roll your shoulders forward in a circular motion five times, then roll them backward five times.

3. **Overhead Arm Stretch:** Raise your arms overhead and interlace your fingers. Lean to the right and hold for 15 seconds, then lean to the left and hold for 15 seconds.

4. **Standing Forward Bend:** Stand with your feet hip-width apart. Bring your arms up to straighten the spine then hinge at your hips and slowly bend forward, reaching for your toes or letting your hands rest in the air or on the floor. Keep your knees slightly bent if needed. Hold for 20 seconds, feeling the stretch in your hamstrings and lower back.

5. **Standing Quad** Stretch: Stand on your left leg and bend your right knee, bringing your heel toward your buttocks. Grab your right ankle

with your right hand, keeping your knees close together. Hold for 15 seconds, then switch legs.

If you have a bit of extra time and the environment allows this, add two more seated stretches.

1. **Seated Forward Bend:** Sit on the floor with your legs extended straight. Slowly reach for your toes, keeping your back straight. Hold for 20 seconds, feeling the stretch in your hamstrings and lower back.

2. **Seated Twist:** Sit with your legs extended. Bend your right knee and place your foot on the outside of your left thigh. Twist your torso to the right, placing your left elbow on the outside of your right knee for leverage. Hold for 15 seconds, then repeat on the other side.

In case you don't want to do this alone, I often recommend one of the leading yoga teachers worldwide, Mady Morrison, to my clients. Her YouTube channel has over 3.5 million followers, and she has a beautiful full-body stretch routine. Through the gentle stretches, we can activate our cores, our sides, our lower backs and spines, our upper torsos, chests and shoulders—parts of the body that are assumed to hold more trauma than other parts.

While therapists and scientists are beginning to agree on the fact that our bodies somehow save and remember painful, difficult or traumatic events, there is still too little research to really know for sure where and how trauma is stored in the body. Also, some people are convinced that most of the trauma is stored in the hips. The logical explanation is that the psoas muscle is largely involved in the fight-or-flight activation of the legs. Having had yoga and yoga therapy as a big influential factor in my personal healing journey, I personally do not see established research to be convinced. Either way, just give the stretching a try, even if it helps with nothing more than making you feel a bit more connected to your body and it invites a gentle activation.

Why not stretch every day for the next 7 days? You can make this part of your morning routine right after you wake up. And remember, you don't have to do this alone; you can be guided by a professional at absolutely no cost.

11. Weightlifting

Generally, these light movements and exercises helped all of my clients gradually move out of dorsal vagal shut-down. It may have taken time for some, but eventually a combination of the movements used together with talk therapy worked. Not in the case of my client, Carrie, though. With Carrie, I tried the majority of the described tools, yet nothing seemed to work. After 6 sessions, I started to become a bit desperate, as Carrie was in dorsal vagal shut-down from our first session. She would say to herself, "I just feel so incredibly stuck, like there is no possible way to get out of this situation." I contemplated asking a colleague whether he would feel comfortable continuing to work with her. He said he would, but felt that was not needed at the time. I explained a bit of the situation, including everything that I had tried, and how I was a bit at the end of my wits. He said, "Have you sent her to the gym to lift?"

I answered, "Have I done what?" Of course, I always suggest that my clients exercise and increase their movement when they are stuck in dorsal vagal shut-down. But I wouldn't specifically send them to the gym. He mentioned that he had recently read an article about how lifting weights makes your nervous system stronger, and that he had started recommending it to some of his clients, specifically those stuck in dorsal vagal shut-down.[16] He made sure to tell them to lift light to medium weights (not more), and that he began to see changes with all of his clients in one or two sessions.

I was intrigued and gave my client Carrie the same advice. She loved to go on long nature walks and was generally a movement advocate, but she had never joined a gym, nor had she ever lifted weights to train different parts of the body. She joined a gym in her neighborhood, got herself a personal trainer, and within four sessions, I could feel a change in her entire being when she came to see me. Her body was no longer flappy, lacking body tension, but more firm and erect. She generally seemed more present and less lost in her mind and her thoughts. She reported that she'd had moments of really feeling herself and had even started to cry during one of the workout sessions. I encouraged her to keep it up and just be gentle with increasing weights or intensifying training. Within a couple of months, we were able to really address and work through some of her major topics for the first time.

Now if you think to yourself that you don't have the money to join a gym, or there is no gym where you live, that's ok. You can just get yourself a pair of dumbbells between 3–5 kg, or 5-10 lbs. Again, you can find so much inspiration for exercises online. Or even better, most of us have that one friend who is an exercise freak who practically lives at the gym, and has been waiting for the day to introduce us to weightlifting for years.

12. Listening to Invigorating Music

Listening to invigorating music can help you or your clients come out of the dorsal vagal shutdown response by engaging the nervous system, boosting positive emotions and fostering a sense of connection and safety. Upbeat music can activate the autonomic nervous system, increasing arousal and energy levels, which counters the low-energy state associated with dorsal vagal shut-down. This can help shift the body from a state of immobilization to one of engagement and readiness. Moreover, enjoyable music triggers the release of dopamine, a neurotransmitter linked to pleasure and reward. Higher dopamine levels improve mood and motivation, helping lift individuals out of depressive or immobilized states. Studies have demonstrated that music-induced dopamine release can significantly enhance feelings of pleasure and motivation.[17] In fact, music therapy is a recognized and legitimate form of therapy that can fill entire books.

Here is a short practice I am inviting you to: Read the instructions below or listen to the guided audio for the exercise accessible by scanning the following QR code or using this url: *https://bit.ly/ptmadesimple*

1. **Choose Your Music:** Select invigorating and upbeat music that you enjoy.

2. **Create a Comfortable Space:** Find a quiet, comfortable place where you can sit or lie down without distractions.

3. **Use Headphones:** For an immersive experience, use headphones to fully engage with the music.

4. **Focus on the Music:** Close your eyes and take deep breaths to relax. Focus on the rhythm, melody and lyrics, allowing yourself to be fully absorbed in the sound.

5. **Move to the Beat:** If you feel inclined, let your body move to the music, such as tapping your feet, nodding your head, or dancing.

6. **Reflect:** After listening, notice how you feel. Are you more energized? Do you feel more present and connected?

Incorporate this practice into your daily routine, especially during stressful times. Regularly engaging with invigorating music can help maintain a balanced and resilient nervous system.

13. Getting Out in the Sun

Dr. Stephen Porges emphasizes the importance of sensory experiences in regulating the nervous system. Engaging with pleasant sensory stimuli, such as sunlight, can help shift the nervous system from a state of shutdown to one of safety and connection.[18] On top of that, exposure to natural light stimulates the production of serotonin, a neurotransmitter that enhances mood and promotes feelings of well-being.

It also regulates circadian rhythms, improving sleep quality and energy levels, which are often disrupted during dorsal vagal shut-down. This practice is simple if you have natural sunlight currently available where you live. Remember that you want to avoid very strong sun exposure, so depending on the season and where you live, you may need to practice early in the morning or in the middle of the day.

Here is the practice:

1. **Find a Sunny Spot:** Identify a safe, comfortable outdoor location with ample sunlight.

2. **Daily Practice:** Spend 15–20 minutes in direct sunlight each morning. Early sunlight is preferable for regulating circadian rhythms. Do this for at least 7 days, then continue doing this practice every 2 or 3 days if you find yourself not having enough time. Some form of consistency is key.

3. **Mindful Presence:** While in the sunlight, focus on your breathing. Take slow, deep breaths to calm the nervous system.

4. **Engage the Senses:** Notice the warmth on your skin, the light filtering through the trees, and the surrounding sounds. Engage your senses fully.

5. **Practice Gratitude:** Reflect on something positive, fostering a sense of gratitude and safety.

I hope you found the many practices in this chapter, mainly intended to help you out of dorsal vagal shut-down, to be helpful. It is not always easy to determine whether you or someone that you are working with is currently in this state of feeling frozen or collapsed. To help you, remember that this response can show symptoms at the level of the body, mind or emotions, and that these can be different for every person. Yet, since people usually have less mobility or even feel paralyzed, any form of light to medium movement is generally supportive for moving out of the freeze response. Plus, creating space for feelings of dissociation and numbness while ensuring you are in a safe environment and feel supported, can help the movement up the ladder into sympathetic activation and eventually back into connection and social engagement.

CHAPTER 4

Moving Through Sympathetic Activation

According to the polyvagal theory, when people move out of parasympathetic dorsal vagal shut-down, usually one out of two things happens: either a return to parasympathetic ventral vagal social engagement or, more likely, a stepping into sympathetic activation. Imagine the following scenario: You grow up in a household with unpredictable, emotionally unavailable parents and regularly experience physical violence. Since you are just a child, you do not have the tools and means to protect or defend yourself. Maybe your body goes into fight-or-flight a few times but it quickly gives up and initiates a freeze-or-shut-down response as the only way of protection it knows.

Eventually you grow up, not really realizing that you are living a big part of your life feeling shut down and frozen. Over the course of your life, with the help of supportive friends and a loving partner, you slowly begin to come out of this shut-down response and find yourself feeling much more intensely than you ever have before. All of a sudden, you are fearful, anxious and worried, and you often find yourself getting into arguments and verbal fights. What is happening here? The body is assumed to remember the difficult and traumatic experiences of the past.

When the body may want to react with fight-or-flight but simply cannot or no longer can, it may suppress the activating sympathetic response and initiate a shut-down response instead. When we come out of the shut-down, the body may want and even need to go back to act out the initial sympathetic response. The following section will share with you a series of tools to help you do exactly this. Please take the utmost care when going through the following practices and ensure that you have the mental, emotional and physical stability at this time to be able to do the exercises. If, at any point, you feel overwhelmed or in need of support, please reach out to a licensed professional.

1. Conversations With the Body

Many people struggle when it comes to deciphering the needs of the body. We are taught to ignore and go beyond these needs and suck it up in critical times. My client Jeremy was one of the many I have worked with, who was raised in a family that praised and rewarded exactly this kind of behavior - to keep going and never show any sign of tiredness, exhaustion or emotion. Jeremy was a father of two beautiful little girls, the provider for the family, and an internationally recognized triathlete.

In his late 40s, after his business unexpectedly grew after he and his family re-settled in Europe, Jeremy started having chest pains during the day and difficulty sleeping at night. Out of nowhere, he started to feel anxious in public spaces and even found himself having a panic attack before an important client meeting. He wasn't the first person I had supported through these kinds of topics, and when Jeremy came to me, I knew that his body had had enough of being ignored and pushed, and was once again simply doing what it does best: ensuring Jeremy's survival. The symptoms were a clear sign from the body saying "I am tired," and "It's enough."

If we don't listen to our bodies, they will find a way to make us listen. When Jeremy came to me for the first time, I started asking him what he was feeling, where he was, and what he thought his body might need. Asking him these questions was like asking a toddler about quantum physics. It was absolutely impossible for him to respond to any of my questions. So I knew I had to slowly help Jeremy get back into connection with his body. Since he was very reflective and mentally strong, I had a feeling that a practice I call " Conversations With the Body" would help. Read the instructions below or listen to the guided audio for this exercise accessible by scanning the following QR code or using this url: *https://bit.ly/ptmadesimple*

- Do this practice when you are wearing some comfortable and loose clothing. You will want to feel as relaxed as you possibly can. Of course, you can also do this practice in sympathetic activation, but it may be easier to practice and become better at this when you are not feeling anxious, agitated, worried or angry.

- Gently shake out the body to begin. As with basically all of these practices, take a deep breath to begin. Do this especially if you are feeling agitated or angry.

- See if you can come to stand still with both feet firmly planted on the ground and start scanning your body to see where you can find an activation. Name the areas where you feel an activation. Then answer the following three questions.

  - What does the activation feel like? Find at least three adjectives to describe the activation.

  - If the activation would be able to express itself in words, how would it express itself? What do you think it would want to say?

  - If the activation would be able to express itself in actions, how would it express itself? What do you think it would do?

- Continue scanning your body and answering all three questions for each activation.

- Take a moment to journal any insights after the practice.

Remember that any activation, sensation, emotion or feeling is not in itself bad or uncomfortable. It is your interpretation of the activation that gives it its respective meaning. So, creating conversations in the body is a great way to actually come back to the original meaning of a specific physical sensation or activation. It's a form of detective work that involves figuring out the non-verbal language of the body. What is actually innate and comes naturally can, through trauma or conditioning, simply get lost.

2. Completing the Unfinished Action

In the previous practice, you were asked to tap into your body by feeling into it and creating conversations with it. For some people, this might be super intuitive and easy, others may need to put the workbook down for a minute until they are in the right headspace to be open to having conversations with the body. I know it's a bit out there, but complex challenges require creative solutions. Becoming more receptive and open to the messages of our bodies can feel strange, challenging and overwhelming to begin, but it is something that is crucial to your healing path. On top of that, it can enable a much richer experience of life, all of its facets, diverse experiences and emotions.

If you read the introduction to this chapter, then you will have been reminded of the body's self-protective mechanism to go into shut-down and suppress, and that eventually it needs to feel and potentially express the way it originally wanted to. We will focus on this more in detail using very specific tools later in this chapter. If you were able to answer the third question in the previous exercise (If the activation would be able to express itself in actions, how would it express itself?

What do you think it would do?) with a specific answer, write this answer down here:

_____

_____

_____

_____

Now take just 2–3 seconds and ask yourself if you feel comfortable to act out the needs of the body in this way? Go with the first spontaneous answer and act accordingly. Likely this answer is still "no" and that is okay. If the answer is a relatively confident "yes" and you can ensure that neither you nor anyone else will get hurt or put in danger in any way, go ahead and perform any desired action of the body. Take good care to watch for any symptoms of an overwhelm or freeze response. An example of such an action could just be the clenching of the fists, lying down and hugging your legs or punching a pillow. It can be a very simple, one-step action. If you don't feel comfortable acting out the needs of the body in this way or don't have a clear message from the body yet, that's ok. Be patient and continue on with the practice.

3. Navigating the Intensity

The difficulty with allowing and going into sympathetic activation is, for most people, with navigating the intensity. Remember that your body is preparing itself to fight or flee as blood rushes to your limbs. The heart beats faster, and the senses are sharpened. These and many other symptoms of a sympathetic response can feel quite strong and even overwhelming. You may think to yourself, "This is simply too much, and I need to end this." If this is the case, it's okay.

Remember, it is always about moving with compassion and at your own speed. Still, a certain level of intensity is part of a sympathetic response. Without the extra activation of the body and senses, you wouldn't be ready to fight or flee.

Remember, as we are moving up the ladder and back into parasympathetic ventral vagal response, the importance lies in allowing the sensations and emotions that we were not able to feel or express when the event actually happened. Depending on the situation and our capacity to cope with the intensity, we will all react differently.

Let's find a way for you to be able to quantify the intensity of the experiences. This will help you determine whether it's safe for you to continue a practice alone, come back later or seek professional support. Take a look at the scale on the next page and mark the intensity of your perceived experience.

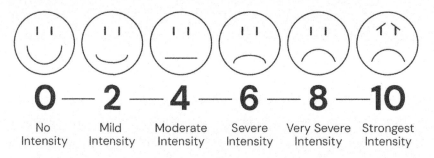

0	2	4	6	8	10
No Intensity	Mild Intensity	Moderate Intensity	Severe Intensity	Very Severe Intensity	Strongest Intensity

How you perceive the intensity of a sympathetic activation is highly dependent on you. When using this scale and rating an experience according to its intensity, two people may state something completely different. Also, for some, an experience of a mild intensity may be too much to handle alone, while for others it may require an experience of very severe intensity before they need support. For this reason, I am not giving a specific recommendation for you on when to work by yourself and when to involve a professional. Decide for yourself now what level of intensity you feel comfortable handling by yourself and when you will consider getting support.

4. Expanding Your Window of Tolerance

Dan Siegel introduced the concept of the "window of tolerance," which refers to the optimal range of emotional arousal within which individuals can function effectively. This range varies for each person and can be significantly influenced by trauma and challenging life experiences. Beyond this window, there are two other states: hypoarousal and hyperarousal. The window of tolerance determines whether we respond to situations with curiosity, openness, presence, flexibility and emotional stability, or if we fall into hypoarousal (characterized by shutting down, numbness, withdrawal, shame and disconnection) or hyperarousal (marked by high energy, anger, panic, anxiety, overwhelm, a fight-or-flight response and chaos).[19] You may see the connection with PVT and the three responses of the nervous system (1. Ventral vagal social engagement 2. Dorsal vagal shut-down and 3. Sympathetic response).

The Window of Tolerance

Hyper Arousal
Fight and flight. Increased heart rate. Agitation. Fear. Anger. Lack of safety

Optimal State: Feeling Safe
Rest and digest. Socially engaged. Calm. Connected. At ease. Creative.

Hypo Arousal
Immobilised. Quiet. Collapsed. Numb. Heavy. Despairing. Zoning out.

Let's practice expanding your window of tolerance. First, take a moment to reflect on your current window of tolerance. Take some time to think about what is generally inside and outside your window of tolerance. See if you can simply observe what situations, people or experiences are part of this window and which ones are not. Then we will do a short practice with the aim of expanding your window of tolerance. Please note that this practice may cause some discomfort.

1. **Preparation:** Move your body to loosen up. Stretch or shake out your body.

2. **Begin:** Sit comfortably, close your eyes, and take a few deep breaths. If closing your eyes is difficult, look at a spot on the ground with unfocused eyes.

3. **Visualize:** Picture your window of tolerance, its size, shape, and the people, situations and events within it.

4. **Expand:** Choose something just outside your current window that might trigger you. Imagine including this in your window for a moment. Choose something of light to medium intensity (max).

5. **Observe:** Notice any sensations, thoughts and emotions. See if you can reduce these symptoms over time.

6. **Safe Space:** If you feel overwhelmed, return to an imagined experience that is well within your window of tolerance. Move between situations or events inside and outside your window of tolerance until it causes fewer reactions.

7. **Repeat:** Continue until you can expand your window without overwhelming symptoms. If it's too intense, take a break.

Finish by relaxing for a few moments thinking of something that you love. Be gentle with yourself as you finish the practice and give your body any love and care it might be asking for afterward.

5. Activation of the Optical Nerve

Remember that moving through and out of sympathetic activation is done by activating the vagus nerve, and therefore activating the parasympathetic nervous system. Many methods were already mentioned here at the beginning of the workbook. Another one I would like to mention at this point is the direct involvement of the optical nerve. Activating this optic nerve can help someone come out of sympathetic activation. One of the simplest practices just involves shifting your gaze or engaging in specific eye movements.

A very simple movement, together with an orienting practice, is to simply turn your head as far back as you can to describe an object that is behind you. You can turn to the left or the right, whichever is more comfortable for you. Turn your head only as far as you can and as long as it still feels comfortable. Remain with the head turned for at least 30 or 60 seconds while describing the object.

This method works because the neck movement stimulates the vagus nerve and other nerves sitting in the cervical region of the spine. Also, simply stretching different body parts—in this case, the neck, can bring a sense of relaxation and calm.

6. The Polar Bear Spasms

Dr. Peter Levine, an American psychologist, trauma expert and best-selling author, made an interesting observation in the behavior of animals, specifically polar bears, in response to being tranquilized. He found that as the bear wakes after the sedation, its body trembles and shakes intensely while making biting motions over the shoulder. After some moments, the bear goes into a deep gasping. Levine explained that the polar bear was completing the fight-flight action it would have likely performed if it were not sedated. Levine saw this as the completion of a trauma response, which he believes is also needed in humans in order to process traumatic events and ensure the intense energy we experienced during the event doesn't get stuck and then makes us sick.[20]

When humans have a traumatic experience, such as a car accident or physical assault, social conditioning, shame and guilt often don't allow us to adequately process the experience. Instead of releasing the built-up tension or fears after an accident through crying, for example, we quickly gather ourselves to exchange contact and insurance details and get out of the way. In a therapeutic setting, people are helped to move through and process the excess energy and stored-up emotions bit by bit.

This workbook is inviting you to do exactly the same, so always remember that when it comes to moving through somatic activation, it is most important to move slowly, with caution and care. You will be invited to release some of the excess energy over the course of the next 10 practices. Also, once you have read through this section, you can go back to doing any of the practices that activate the vagus nerve by using your breath or using touch with the intention of bringing a gradual release.

Before we do this, let's just do a little reflection.

Imagine what this acting out of the fight-or-flight responses can look like in humans. What could we potentially do physically? Contemplate this for a few minutes, and then write down your ideas.

_____

_____

_____

_____

Do you ever remember yourself acting out the sympathetic fight- or flight response after coming out of a parasympathetic collapse or freeze response?

_____

_____

_____

_____

7. Safely Acting Out Fight- or Flight-Response

This practice will invite you into a difficult or traumatic memory, so please only do this at a time when you feel relatively stable and grounded. Otherwise, do this practice with support and guidance. Work with an event of light to medium intensity to begin, and find yourself a safe, comfortable and quiet place for this practice.

Read the instructions below or listen to the guided audio for this exercise accessible by scanning the following QR code or using this url: *https://bit.ly/ptmadesimple*

- Sit or lie down and take a couple of deep belly breaths to begin this practice. Remember, if any intensity arises during the practice, you can re-initiate the deep breathing to help calm the nervous system. But also remember that this exercise is intended to lead you back into experiencing what may have been numbed or suppressed during the actual event. Take about 1-2 minutes to settle into the practice in this way.

- When you feel ready, begin to remember the actual event and anything leading up to it. Take your time and ensure you do not overwhelm yourself with this practice. Just see what comes up as you allow yourself to go back in time, without going into too many stories of the mind or getting carried away by thoughts. Take about 2-3 minutes for this step.

- While continuing to remember the event, begin observing any sensations in your body. What sensations are you perceiving and where? Is there any form of movement that your body would like to make as you experience these sensations? If yes, and it is safe for you, go ahead and make the movement(s). Take your time (roughly 2-4 minutes) doing this and continue feeling the sensations of the body or performing movements the body would like to make.

- Begin to remember how you felt after the event and what you did right after. Is there anything else that you would have wanted to do instead? Are there any emotions that would have been needed to be expressed? See if you feel comfortable expressing any of these emotions verbally. Please ensure that only things that do not put you or anyone else at risk should be expressed or acted out. Again take about 2-4 minutes for this step.

- See how you feel after these minutes of going into the sensations and emotions of the body, and check in for yourself whether you feel you would like to continue a bit longer with the practice. You can do this as many times as you like whenever you feel that there are still movements, words or expressions coming up for that specific event.

- Once the practice feels complete, or you notice a sense of tiredness or fatigue (a sign that our capacity for emotional processing is at its maximum for now), gently stop the practice by taking a few deep breaths. Remember a place where you feel safe and supported, or remember someone you love.

- Journal any insights gained after the practice.

_____

_____

_____

_____

8. Releasing Trauma Through the Physiological Sigh

The "physiological sigh" is a natural breathing pattern that helps reduce stress and anxiety by enhancing oxygen levels and stimulating the parasympathetic nervous system. This breathing technique involves two inhales through the nose followed by a long exhale through the mouth. This technique can help reduce stress and manage the body's sympathetic activation, which is often heightened in individuals experiencing trauma.[21] The practice activates the parasympathetic nervous system, promoting relaxation and aiding in the release of stored trauma.

Here is a short practice of the physiological sigh:

1. Find a comfortable position sitting or lying down.

2. Take a deep breath in through your nose, filling your lungs completely.

3. Immediately following the first inhale, take a second, shorter inhale to fully expand the air sacs in your lungs. Here is where oxygen and carbon dioxide are exchanged.

4. Then exhale slowly and fully through your mouth, extending the exhalation as long as possible.

5. Perform 3–5 physiological sighs.

6. Continue breathing naturally and feel into any effects of this practice.

The physiological sigh can help reduce heart rate and anxiety, critical for managing stress and releasing trauma. Regular practice helps shift the nervous system toward calmness and safety, facilitating emotional regulation and healing.

9. Shaking to Aid the Release

Maybe you did the last practices, and besides getting quite emotional and pulled back into old memories and negative patterns of thinking, not much happened. You did the practices according to the instructions, but there were no sensations that you were feeling in the body or any movements that wanted to be acted out. This is quite normal, as moving out of dorsal vagal shut-down into sympathetic activation and release is not a straight-forward process that will always move from point A to B.

Sometimes you might move into a little sympathetic activation, and the moment you do this, your brain sends an alarm response, and you go immediately back into shut-down. You might be moving back and forth between these states a few times throughout the day or through practice. If you do feel that the sympathetic activation seems to have passed at some point or that you are simply not feeling enough of it, here is a practice that can help you move through sympathetic activation and in some cases increase the intensity of the felt experience to help you go deeper into the memory and the release of stored trauma.

This is a practice that can be both a bit intense and, for some people, a bit physically tiring. So ensure that you have the mental, emotional and physical capacity to practice at this time. Of course, you can also do this practice when you are already experiencing some intensity. In this case, please take good care.

Read the instructions below or listen to the guided audio for this exercise accessible by scanning the following QR code or using this url: *https://bit.ly/ptmadesimple*

Shaking the Body

- Wear loose and comfortable clothing for this practice, and practice on an empty stomach. Before you begin, reflect on your current level of stress, anxiety or agitation from 0 to 10 (0 = no stress, anxiety, or agitation at all, and 10 = maximum stress, anxiety or agitation).

- Begin the practice by gently starting to bounce up and down, bending the knees a little, and moving the body up and down.

- Then start incorporating your fingers and hands and begin shaking them lightly as you move the body up and down.

- Over time, start to include the arms and shoulders. And eventually incorporate the feet and the legs.

- Finally, also begin to lightly shake your head.

- With time, you are going to increase the intensity of the shaking all over the body. Continue this practice for 3–5 minutes. If you like, you can also do this practice with invigorating music you enjoy.

- If you feel any emotions, sensations or thoughts arising, it will be as if you are shaking all of this out of your body. If you begin to cry, laugh or even have the impulse to scream, do so while you continue the shaking.

- If things get too much for you at any point, reduce the intensity of shaking a bit and incorporate deeper breaths.

- Take some time to rest afterward. This practice is like doing a workout, to support your mind and your emotions.

10. Tapping to Help Release

For many clients going back into painful and traumatic memories is simply too overwhelming. Also, for many the sympathetic activation and fight- or -flight response is so strong that they immediately go back into dorsal shutdown. My client Eva was such a case. When going back into remembering what had happened to her in one of her previous relationships, she would get so angry that we both weren't sure if she could move through and process her anger in a healthy way. And as someone who supports others in this journey, I need to be sure that what I offer is safe for clients and that whatever Pandora box is opened needs to be adequately processed before I send my clients on their way.

So with Eva I simply couldn't do a lot of the practices that could potentially bring up some intensity. One weekend before our session, I had received an Emotional Freedom Technique (EFT) session from a friend in which very strong negative emotions came up for me. I was almost a bit shocked, not realizing I was holding so much frustration and anger related to a specific person inside of me. The session was virtual, so my friend and therapist started guiding me through different tapping points, while I would repeat certain statements.

Within minutes the intensity was manageable and I noticed that I became much calmer. Then my therapist guided me back into the specific memory and situation, and again quite intense emotions of anger and frustration came up, just a bit weaker this time. Again, I did a few rounds of tapping while I repeated some phrases. It seems that the mental preoccupation (through the sentences) and the physical tapping really supported me in being with and eventually moving through the emotions. After a few rounds the associated feelings were still there but not to a point where they were really bothering me. I took this as inspiration into my next session with Eva and decided to do the following self-guided EFT practice with her.

EFT is often facilitated by a trained professional, but it can also be practiced independently. Here's is a short guide to such a practice:

Begin by formulating the sentence that you will be asked to repeat.

- Identify the source of distress, such as physical discomfort, emotions or challenging thoughts.

- Assess the intensity of the issue on a scale from 0 to 10.

- Craft a statement such as: "Even though I have this _____ _____ , I deeply and completely accept myself and how I feel."

- Tap the fleshy part on the side of your hand underneath the pinky finger with two or more fingers while repeating the statement. Continue repeating the statement while tapping on 8 specific acupoints (see the diagram).

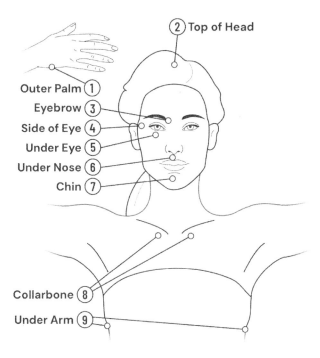

- After each cycle, evaluate the intensity of the issue. Repeat the process 2–3 times or until notable relief is achieved.

- Reflect on your emotions and experiences in a journal after practicing.

11. Reducing Stress Through Visual Stimulation: Fractals

When we are in a state of sympathetic activation, calming our nervous systems is sometimes easier than we think. An extremely powerful, yet simple method is introducing specific visual stimulation, through showing actual objects or using our imaginations. There are many different approaches to this, and I would like to spend the next few tools elaborating on some of the most effective ones. Let's begin by practicing using actual visual stimulation using fractals.

Fractals are geometric figures with repeating patterns. They are everywhere, and you can find them when taking a close look at a leaf, a piece of art, or even a building. The University of Oregon actually found that looking at fractals can reduce stress by 60%.[22] It seems that somehow, fractals have a hypnotic and calming effect on us. It's important to pick a fractal that doesn't trigger any negative or traumatic memories, which is why I recommend working with black and white fractals for patients with PTSD, C-PTSD, or trauma.

The practice: Pick one of the two fractals following these instructions that you resonate with most. Don't give it too much thought and just pick the one that feels most interesting and inspiring to look at. Find yourself a comfortable space, ideally sitting down. Begin to look at the fractal. First, look at it as a whole, then begin to explore the details of the fractal.

Once you have quenched your curiosity about exploring the details, continue looking at the image with more of an unfocused view. Continue this practice for about 3–5 minutes. The whole practice can take up to 5–7 minutes. I know this is quite a long time to look at a geometric image, but why not give it a try? If you find this practice to be very supportive, you can print out your favorite fractal, laminate it and carry it with you. Such a practice can easily be done in the office or on any public transport. It's absolutely free and for many people it is very effective!

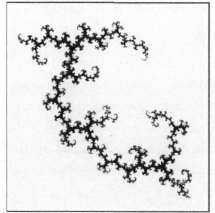 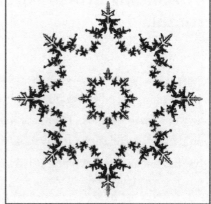

Journal any insights gained after the practice.

Note: Looking at fractals can create dizziness or nausea for some people. If this is the case, the same practice can be done using a picture or photograph from a beautiful scene in nature. If this is done in real life it's even more effective, as you will have the full sensory experience of sight, sound, smell and even touch.

12. Reducing Stress Through Visual Stimulation: Guided Visualization of Your Safe Space

In *Chapter 1 Practice # 7* I shared with you simple mindfulness meditation to help activate the vagus nerve and create a state of calm and relaxation. Here is a similar practice of doing a guided visualization to help you feel more at ease. Please note that if you or a client is experiencing any kind of traumatic flashbacks or memories, it is better to work with actual visual objects rather than imagination, as closing the eyes in those cases can intensify what someone is internally experiencing.

If you have practiced this method before while experiencing sympathetic activation of the difficult memories, it can be used with care and ideally with guidance. If you are currently experiencing symptoms of anxiety, not feeling grounded or connected with yourself or even feeling a sense of helplessness, the following technique can be quite supportive. Remember that it is fully up to you to try a specific technique and then decide for yourself whether this technique is supportive for you or not. If not, don't worry. You can find almost 70 alternative practices in this workbook to choose from.

If you feel ready to be guided into your safe space, read the instructions below or listen to the guided audio for this exercise accessible by scanning the following QR code or using this url: *https://bit.ly/ptmadesimple*

- Close your eyes and take a deep breath. Remain like this for some moments, breathing deeply and just focusing on relaxing your body, emotions and mind.

- Become aware of the present moment, and how tension and anxiety may decrease by connecting with the here and now. If it works, great! If not, that's also ok. Release expectations and ideas about this practice.

- When you feel ready, begin to imagine a place where you feel completely safe and at ease. This can be any place that brings a sense of protection and support. Just see what your mind begins to create in front of your inner eye as you imagine your safe space.

- Your safe space could be a quiet beach with gentle waves, a serene forest with rustling leaves and dappled sunlight or a cozy room with a crackling fire and a snug blanket, just to mention some examples.

- Picture yourself in this safe space, surrounded by these comforting sights, sounds and scents. Feel the ground beneath you, whether it's soft sand, cool grass or a comfortable chair.

- In this space, you are completely supported and at peace. Remain in this space for as long as you like. Remain until you feel more calm and more at peace.

- Whenever you feel ready, begin to slowly leave this place, coming back into the here and now, perceiving the noises that surround you and eventually and slowly opening your eyes.

- Whenever you need to find calm and safety, remember that you can return to this special place in your mind.

Calming visualizations can trigger the parasympathetic nervous system, allowing your body to feel genuinely relaxed. You can also do this practice by traveling to places where you once felt at peace. Hopefully this practice allowed you to experience a few quiet moments.

Do you prefer using actual objects or your imagination for the visualization practices? Why?

_____

_____

_____

_____

13. Reducing Stress Through Visual Stimulation: Visual Stimulation and Breathing

If you have read through the other parts of the workbook, surely you remember the series of breathing practices I introduced in Chapter 1. When you become comfortable at both the breathing and visual stimulation practices, you can begin combining these. As you can imagine, combining these practices can be even more effective. Ensure that you feel comfortable with the deep belly breathing in Chapter 1 before you continue on with this practice.

Read the instructions below or listen to the guided audio for this exercise accessible by scanning the following QR code or using this url:
https://bit.ly/ptmadesimple

1. Sit or lie down in a comfortable position in a quiet place where you won't be disturbed.

2. Gently close your eyes and take a few moments to settle in. Allow your body to relax.

3. Begin the deep belly breathing:

   - Inhale deeply through your nose, filling your lungs and then belly completely.

   - See how your belly gently expands as you inhale.

   - Begin to slowly exhale all the air through the mouth, gently contracting the abdominal muscles to release all the air.

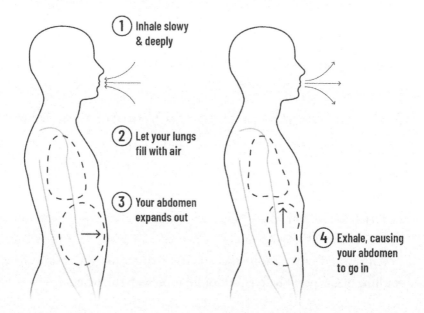

4. Continue this deep breathing pattern for several minutes, focusing on the rhythm of your breath.

5. As you continue deep breathing, imagine yourself in your safe space. This could be the same space from the previous practice or a serene

beach, a tranquil forest, or any place where you feel safe and relaxed. Picture every detail of this place. Visualize the colors, the light and the textures around you.

6. Imagine all the sounds you would hear in this place, such as waves gently crashing, birds chirping or leaves rustling in the wind. Visualize the scents you would smell, like salty sea air, fresh pine or blooming flowers. Feel the sensations on your skin, such as the warmth of the sun, a cool breeze or the softness of the ground beneath you.

7. With each breath, deepen the visualizations and your connection to this peaceful place. Allow yourself to feel more and more relaxed and at ease.

8. If your mind starts to wander, gently bring your focus back to your breath and the vivid details of your visualized setting.

9. Slowly conclude the practice after about 7–10 minutes by gradually bringing your awareness back to the present moment. Notice how and where you are sitting or laying down, while wiggling your fingers and toes. Eventually, open your eyes and notice the room in which you are, taking note of any sights, sounds or smells in the present moment.

10. Take a few moments to reflect on how you feel. Appreciate the sense of calm and relaxation you have created.

If you enjoyed this breathing and visualization practice, why not do this meditation for the next seven days before you go to sleep?

14. The Sounds You Enjoy

What are some sounds you really enjoy listening to? For most people, certain types of sounds are very calming. For some, it's the chirping of birds; for others, it's exotic jungle sounds, and many people really enjoy listening to the waves of the ocean or rainfall. But not only nature sounds are soothing in this way. More examples include: soft music, like classical or instrumental without lyrics, or gentle animal sounds such as the purring of cats.

Surely you have sat by a bonfire or fireplace at some point, and really enjoyed the crackling of the wooden logs? Or what about the sound of wind chimes? Surely you feel a resonance with one of these examples.

Here is another category of sounds that you may not have heard of yet: The so-called ASMR sounds. ASMR, or autonomous sensory meridian response, is a term used to describe a tingling sensation that typically begins on the scalp and moves down the back of the neck and spine. This sensation is often triggered by specific auditory or visual stimuli, such as soft whispering, tapping or gentle hand movements. Even the crinkling of paper or plastic, or the sounds of brushing hair, can trigger ASMR for some people. ASMR trigger sounds are produced and recorded while using high-quality mics, and then can support millions of listeners with relaxation, focus and even sleep. They have become so popular over the past few years that YouTube content creators are entirely living off of the millions of subscribers that regularly listen to their recordings.

The sounds we enjoy that soothe us are highly individual, of course. From a scientific perspective, music therapy has been proven to be effective in reducing anxiety and depression.[23] Other studies have found that nature sounds significantly reduce stress.[24] So in case you are not working with music as a safe and easy way to help you calm your nervous system and return to a state of parasympathetic activation yet, I would highly suggest that you give this a try.

Decide now whether you would like to listen to different nature sounds (such as sounds of water or of birds), classical or instrumental music, or try ASMR sounds. You can find professional recordings on YouTube and also on yoga and meditation apps such as Calm or InsightTimer. Much of the content is also available free of charge on these apps. Just search for one of the above-mentioned categories and find a track of 3–7 minutes.

Once you have found a track, just listen to it for a few seconds and see if it generally resonates. If a track generally resonates, just pick it and begin listening. There is no right or wrong here, and you have other days and opportunities to try something else. Ensure that you have a quiet and calm space, ideally for yourself. Get comfortable sitting or lying down.

As you begin listening to the track, try to relax as much as possible and fully immerse yourself in the sounds and the recording. Allow the sounds and music to move through your body, a bit like it is activating all the cells in your body. Feel the music in your whole body until the recording ends. Then take a few minutes to rest in silence, feeling the effects of this practice. Note carefully how you feel before and after. Journal about this experience, any insights and how you feel before and after.

---

15. Dancings Emotions

Sympathetic activation is often characterized by strong sensations and emotions. Many of the tools in this chapter focus on learning to be with and releasing strong emotions or sensations through some form or movement and/or really tapping into and expressing what is being felt. For most people, really tapping into what is alive emotionally and physically is often overwhelming. We are simply not taught to allow our feelings and emotions to be felt, and surely not expressed in such ways. So it makes perfect sense that feelings and emotions overwhelm us. If then paired with experiences of trauma or other mental health challenges, emotions and sensations become even more overwhelming.

So for most people, really experiencing and authentically, yet safely, expressing their emotions becomes a life-long journey. Expressing our emotions is not easy, and none of the practices in this chapter are suggesting that it is. If we don't learn about our personal triggers and what causes specific emotional reactions, we will be at the mercy of these and they will determine the course of our lives. Emotions are known to literally hijack our brains, so the best thing we can do is catch them in a state of light to medium intensity before they have fully taken over.

But what if things have begun to spiral and you feel your emotions getting out of control? Earlier practices in this chapter suggest different kinds of movements, like doing some exercise and even going to the gym to lift weights. There is also another alternative, which for most people would be considered much more fun. Surely you have guessed it already due to the title. It is "dancing your emotions". Many, if not to say most people, actually like to dance. If you take away being watched and potentially judged by others, and also judging yourself, most people will naturally begin to move their bodies as their favorite song begins to play. If no one was watching (and judging), we would probably all enjoy dancing, as long as our bodies would allow this. So this practice invites you into exactly this: a space where you can invite your body to simply express itself in whichever way it likes.

A practice where the mind-body connection can be strengthened through the intuitive movements done, as difficult and even traumatic memories arise. Please ensure you do this practice with the support of a licensed professional, or with the support of someone you really trust and feel supported by. At the same time doing such a practice on your own could allow for a more unfiltered expression of movements, representing what is alive inside. When we know someone is watching, many of us tend to slightly alter our behaviors.

Read the instructions below or listen to the guided audio for this exercise accessible by scanning the following QR code or using this url: *https://bit.ly/ptmadesimple*

- Choose a quiet, comfortable area where you have plenty of space to move freely without interruptions or needing to worry about being seen. Select music that resonates with your current mood or that you know touches you in some way. For example, if you feel angry or upset, see if you can find music that makes you emotional or pick something powerful and rhythmic like drumming or intense instrumental pieces. Examples include Taiko drumming or Hans Zimmer's "Inception" soundtrack. The type of music you choose is really up to you, and if you are doing this practice for the first time and aren't sure, why not practice with a friend or practice using less intense music at first to create less intensity.

- Make sure you are wearing comfortable clothes, come to stand in the middle of the room and close your eyes, and take a few deep breaths. Feel your feet underneath you, anchoring yourself firmly on the ground, remembering that you can pause the practice at any point and time and return to feeling the ground underneath you.

- Begin to play the music and slowly scan your body from head to toe, noticing any areas of tension or discomfort. Breathe into these areas, inviting relaxation.

- Then start with gentle, fluid movements, like shaking your hands, rolling your shoulders and swaying your hips. Allow any tension to flow out through these movements, guided by the rhythm of the music.

- Allow the body to begin moving naturally in whichever way it would like. Try to focus on simply feeling the body and inviting it to move in the way it likes. It doesn't matter what a movement looks like, if it's fluid or synchronized with the music. It's about expressing yourself completely authentically.

- Continue feeling into the body and see if it would like to express an emotion or sensation in any way. You can even ask your body: "Dear body, would you like to express any of the emotions that you are experiencing through specific movements?"' Create movements that symbolize this feeling—perhaps reaching out symbolizes longing, or curling inward represents protection. Let your body naturally express these symbols in sync with the music.

- Give your body time to respond, allow for pauses and again and again deepen the connection to simply feel within. The mind will likely comment something along the lines of "What you are doing?" or become active at certain parts. If this is the case, just come back into your body and into feeling.

- Transition into free-form dancing, combining grounding, making symbolic movements and, if available, releasing emotions and memories from the body. Move intuitively, following your body's impulses and the flow of the music.

- After 10–15 minutes, slow down and return to stillness. Sit or lie down, close your eyes, and take a few deep breaths. Reflect on how you feel and any insights that emerged.

How was this practice for you?

_____

_____

_____

_____

16. Do Absolutely Nothing

I would like to end this chapter on practices to help return to parasympathetic ventral vagal response with probably the most challenging, yet long-term, most effective practice: the practice of doing absolutely nothing when sympathetic activation arises. No matter if this activation comes in the form of anxiety, anger, resentment, pain or any kind of bodily sensation, the challenge is to simply do nothing. Before you call me crazy, here is why: Maybe you have heard the saying "neurons that fire together, wire together," or "where the attention goes, the energy flows." Both statements explain the same idea: Whatever we give attention to will somehow eventually become bigger.

If we experience anger and constantly feed that anger by going back into the stories that make us angry, we are likely to become more and more upset. If we feel sad and heartbroken about a breakup and continue to play our favorite love songs while reminiscing in happy memories with that person, we will probably become more and more sad. Doing nothing breaks the cycle of feeding a thought, an emotion or a sensation. Of course, this doesn't work instantly, but over time it will.

Doing nothing or non-reactivity is a key element of any mindfulness meditation. If you simply stop reacting to the trigger, the trigger will go away over time. Please note that this practice is challenging for most people, as many of us simply cannot deal with the intensity of what is arising within and have to react in some way. Still, non-reactivity can be trained and practiced, and over the course of your life, it will probably become one of your biggest superpowers. Are you up for the challenge to give this a try and train yourself in non-reactivity? If yes, then let's do a very short practice:

Whatever emotions, sensations or thoughts you are experiencing at this moment, I invite you to not react in any way, shape or form. Let the phenomenon arise and be there, and simply see it and watch it. It will be as though you are looking down at whatever is happening from above. If you feel anger or frustration, simply watch these emotions without saying or doing anything. Let them be, without fighting them. See if you and the emotions can somehow co-exist. The same goes for any sensations or difficult thoughts. Allow and accept everything. I know this can be quite tricky, but I also know that you can do this! It only requires one time of not reacting to an emotion, sensation or thought to begin to break our automated responses.

If you do feel at some point that things are just getting too much, and you need to react in some way, I invite you to do the so-called valsalva maneuver. Here, you simply pinch your nose while trying to exhale against the closed airway, keeping your mouth closed. This increases the pressure inside your chest cavity, thereby stimulating your vagus nerve. This method can be used for many different purposes, e.g., to normalize middle ear pressure, for cardiological diagnosis, for strength training, or the regulation of heart rhythm. In this case, it simply activates the vagus nerve, encouraging a parasympathetic activation. On top of that, it creates a momentary distraction that can bring a short form of relief.

You have reached the end of this Chapter where we explored many different practices to help you out of sympathetic activation. As difficult as the experience of sympathetic states such as anxiety, agitation, fears or anger may be, from the standpoint of Stephen Porges and the polyvagal theory, this activation is good and actually needed as you heal from difficult experiences and even trauma from the past. You can see the movement from parasympathetic freeze or collapse to sympathetic activation, like something is being released within you. Stored memories and even trauma that the body somehow saved and still remembers are being stirred up, potentially causing agitation and overwhelm.

Yet the process of stirring things up is generally needed for the mental, emotional and physical processing of experiences we were not able to process properly at the time they happened. So even when somatic activation might feel like things are getting worse, I invite you to trust that whatever is arising has its purpose in wanting to be seen and felt. Moving from somatic activation back into parasympathetic rest and digest (the top of the ladder, according to Deb Dana) is like climbing a high mountain: Somewhere in the middle, you feel so tired, exhausted and overwhelmed that you think you will never make it. If you keep going past that point at whatever speed you can, learn to keep going, learn to safely move through the emotions, fears and overwhelm, then suddenly you will end up at the top.

After 15 minutes of rest at the top, the struggles of the climb already seem very much in the past. Maybe it even seems like it was never that bad. Since the climb to the top can be hard to endure, especially when we walk on our own, let's explore one last chapter in this workbook on how you can walk your healing path according to the polyvagal theory with others: Let's explore PVT, social connection and the ideas behind co-regulation.

PART 4

Polyvagal Theory and Social Connection

Humans are not meant to walk on this earth alone. Since the beginning of time, humans have gathered in groups for support, survival and social connection. Even if you don't consider yourself to be very social, just contemplate for a moment those times in your life where you felt more at ease, maybe even at peace with yourself. It is likely that during those times, you were also seeking or engaged in some form of social connections. And if you think back on the times when you did not feel very happy or very connected to yourself, you might find that you were avoiding or even escaping social connections. Of course, each one of us has different needs and tendencies in terms of wanting to be around others, yet research confirms that people who are more connected to others and have strong social connections live a happier and longer life![25] Also, many psychological illnesses actually have a disruption of social behavior as a core symptom. Just think about depression, anxiety, autism or different kinds of personality disorders.[26]

So what is co-regulation, and why is it important for healing from trauma, PTSD, C-PTSD and many other psychological challenges and illnesses? Co-regulation is the automatic process of our nervous system regulating itself with the nervous systems of those around us. Imagine coming into a room where a befriended couple is arguing heavily. You felt happy, light and excited to see your friends, yet the moment you step into the room, your mood suddenly shifts. You feel uncomfortable, anxious and out of place. Maybe you even feel like turning around right then and there and meeting your friends at another time.

While you were on your way and walking in nature, your brain and nervous system signaled to you that you were safe and that you could relax. The moment you entered the room, your brain and nervous system picked up all these different verbal and nonverbal cues within seconds and activated your sympathetic nervous system. If you grew up in an unsafe environment with lots of shouting, fighting and maybe even physical aggression, a situation like this might also send you straight into a parasympathetic freeze.

As you stay in the room with your friends, and they continue to argue and shout, your body is likely to actually take on the stress and tension of your friends. Nervous systems tend to harmonize and align with each other, and what is moving one person near you is likely to affect you in some way. The neurological correlates of this alignment of our emotional, physical and mental state are the so-called mirror neurons in our brain.[27] They are responsible for exactly what their name implies, mirroring others in their feelings, words and actions.

We learn to co-regulate and mirror others as infants very early on in life through our relationships with our parents and caregivers. If we are met with warm, responsive and consistent interactions as babies, we learn that being around others is safe and can actually help us self-regulate. If we grew up around caregivers who were frequently stressed and anxious and had inconsistent, even unpredictable, interventions with them, our capacity to regulate ourselves in the presence of others is likely to be disturbed. Growing up around someone with a highly dysregulated nervous system can actually change the way you perceive others and the world.

If your parents were living in a state of stress, anxiety, anger or dissociation while you grew up, your nervous system is likely to have taken on their dysregulated state without you needing to have the same experiences that they may have had. And if dysregulation is all you see and know in yourself and those closest to you, you are likely to not even know that how you experience yourself is very different from others. The good news is that even if you grew up in an environment that did not foster connection and therefore failed to help your nervous system learn early on how to regulate itself, this is something that you can learn and practice throughout the course of your life. And the best way to learn how to regulate your nervousness is actually in the presence of others who are themselves regulated.

CHAPTER 5

Return to Ventral Vagal: Tools for Co-regulation and Greater Social Engagement

In this last Chapter we will explore a series of tools supporting you in this process of learning to regulate yourself with and in the presence of others, and help you back into connection with others. You will be invited to reflect on and reach out to those people who you feel you can learn from, and to do a series of partner practices. If you are working with clients, you can use many of these tools directly in your sessions. Remember that your clients are looking to you for orientation and for modeling a regulated nervous system. So no matter if you are actually in a session or accidentally run into a client at a football game or in a bar, be aware of the role you have as a professional to those around you. If you are a client yourself, and are not sure who you can turn to for support at this moment, I will try to offer a few alternatives for partner practices. But do remember co-regulation happens in the presence of others, so even if you do not know at this moment who you can turn to or are scared and anxious to reach out to others, remember that this is a condition of the dysregulated nervous system. The way to healing and completeness is through social connection.

1. Understanding the Idea of Co-Regulation

In case you are not totally sure yet about the idea of co-regulation, let's explore a little practical case to help you understand how co-regulation happens between a child and a caregiver or parent. Take my client Jane, for example. Jane is a very calm and kind woman who is always looking to support others. Over the years she has really been challenged by her oldest son, who started out as a cry baby and is now showing intense frustration and aggression at the age of 5. Jane doesn't have any logical explanation for his behavior, and she tells me from session to session how hard she tries to be a present and supportive mom.

Over the years, she has never lost her temper, but as the behavior is getting more and more extreme, she is a bit at the end of her wits. I explored with her the different tantrums her son is having at home and in public, and finally found a lever that Jane hadn't been putting enough focus on. When Jane's son would act up, I would recommend her to follow these four steps:

1. To stay physically close to her child

2. To stay calm (no matter what was happening for her son)

3. To actually name the feeling or emotion that was behind the behavior of her son

4. To not help until he was ready

Can you guess what step Jane was missing? For Jane, it was step 4. She was such a concerned, supportive and overprotective mom that she would attempt to help her child the moment the tantrum began. Surely out of a fear of her son losing it once again in public, she jumped in, ready to support and console him where needed. Now her son wasn't ready to be helped, as the range of emotions that he was experiencing was still so overwhelming and he needed to move through them first.

Jane needed to learn to be more patient and be able to be in the presence of her son while he was raging. If you have children of your own and have experienced a tantrum, you know this is extremely hard, as the reactions of others trigger a response in our own nervous systems. It is very hard to stay present and calm when someone around us goes into a state of dysregulation, and as I mentioned in the introduction, our nervous systems are actually wired to adapt to one another. This is where you need to stay conscious and aware, both for yourself and for others.

Now think about your own nervous system and a recent tantrum (yes, adults also experience tantrums) you may have had. Now take a look at the 4 steps above. Which of the 4 steps do you find most helpful from others? Why?

_____

_____

_____

_____

Remember a time when someone really supported you and helped you feel calmer and more relaxed?

_____

_____

_____

_____

2. Finding People that Can Help You Co-Regulate

Since we learn how to regulate our own nervous systems from others, one of the most supportive things in your own healing process is being in the presence of others whose nervous systems are mostly regulated. I am saying mostly regulated because I personally do not know of any people that always have themselves and their emotions fully under control. Still, it is very likely that you have people around you that you can learn from.

Write down all the people that you can think of right now that you feel have a regulated or mostly regulated nervous system:

_____

_____

_____

_____

What is something that all these people have in common?

_____

_____

_____

_____

Now take a few more moments to reflect. Who could you imagine being most supported by? Why?

_____

_____

_____

_____

Do you feel this person could be physically, mentally and emotionally available for you at this time?

_____

_____

_____

_____

If not, who is another person from the list you feel inspired to be supported by that is more available?

_____

_____

_____

_____

If you feel inspired, reach out to this person at the end of this practice and find out if there is any kind of support that they are willing and able to offer you at this time. Maybe you can also see if you can be more often in their presence from now on. Remember that just by being around people with a regulated nervous system, your brain unconsciously learns.

3. Survival to Social Engagement Scale

Moving from a dysregulated to a regulated state of the nervous system will always include becoming aware of your state of dysregulation and where you are currently finding yourself on Deb Dana's ladder. In Chapter 3, Practice 2 you can find some guiding questions to help you discover if your nervous system is likely to be dysregulated. Considering you are reading this book, chances are you have and are experiencing some kind of dysregulation.

For this last part on co-regulation and social engagement, please take a look at the following survival to social engagement scale to give you an idea of where you are currently finding yourself on the ladder. You can take a picture of this ladder, print it out and laminate it. Whenever you feel like something is up and you are not fully feeling at ease, take a look at the ladder and see where you are currently at. Count the number of steps you are away from the top (social engagement).

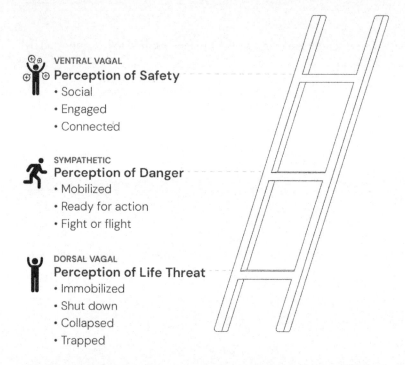

VENTRAL VAGAL
Perception of Safety
- Social
- Engaged
- Connected

SYMPATHETIC
Perception of Danger
- Mobilized
- Ready for action
- Fight or flight

DORSAL VAGAL
Perception of Life Threat
- Immobilized
- Shut down
- Collapsed
- Trapped

4. Practice Activating Mirror Neurons

In regard to co-regulation, I hope the message is clear: You need to surround yourself with people who generally have a regulated nervous system. Of course, it takes time for your nervous system to adjust and align itself with the other person, but with time and some practice, this regulation can happen more quickly. For this reason, therapy or working with a licensed professional becomes crucial for many people with trauma, PTSD and C-PTSD. Co-regulation requires a loving and compassionate presence that you can learn from and whose nervous system you can mirror. A professional will have the most experience and practice supporting you.

While we can learn from others around us, trying to make a close friend or even a partner into your personal therapist not only doesn't work, but is actually unhealthy for the relationship in the long run. So if you are working with others around you, ensure that you remain responsible for your own healing process while respecting others' boundaries. Yet co-regulation can be so simple and much more often experienced than we might realize. Plus, only working with a professional once every few weeks would likely not give you enough exposure to help fully rewire your brain and regulate your nervous system.

Remember the mirror neurons that I talked about in the introduction? Here is one short practice that is based on working on activating the mirror neurons and supporting our nervous system regulation. If you are working with a client, just enact the following behaviors. Use the one you believe works best with your client. If you are a client reading this, ask a friend to support you. This one is not difficult, and anyone can support you with this practice. Ask someone you generally like and enjoy being around.

Yawning time: remember how I shared with you a way to activate the vagus nerve through yawning? Well, if you have ever been around someone who is exhausted and begins to yawn a lot, you know what happens. It takes about 2–3 yawns until you also start yawning. For this practice, simply ask the other person to start yawning around you and pretend that they are really exhausted. They can even say things like, "I am so tired. Oh wow, I need to rest now."

Ask them to keep yawning and see what happens to you. Maybe you notice yourself getting tired and beginning to yawn. If not, practice this one more often. Obviously, you don't want to practice this for so long that you get too sleepy. But if this practice works for you, you can use it from now on to help you get back into parasympathetic ventral vagal response.

Laughing yoga: Laughing yoga, founded by Dr. Madan Kataria in India in 1995, combines laughter exercises with breathing techniques to boost physical and mental well-being. Studies on nurses during the Pandemic have shown that laughing yoga can improve mood, reduce stress and enhance overall health.[28]

Laughing yoga can support you, especially if you are finding yourself in a more neutral or negative mood. If you are currently emotionally, mentally or physically overwhelmed, save this practice for another time. If this is the case for you, practices that invite you into slowly feeling and releasing, or gentle co-regulation through touch, can be more supportive.

Here's how you can practice laughing yoga with a partner:

1. **Warm-Up:**
   - Face your partner, make eye contact, and greet each other with a warm smile.
   - Clap rhythmically (1-2, 1-2-3) while chanting "Ho Ho, Ha Ha Ha."

2. **Breathing Exercise:**
   - Inhale deeply through the nose, hold, and exhale slowly through the mouth. Repeat 3–4 times.

3. **Practice each of the following laughing practices for 1–2 minutes each:**
   - Silent Laughter: Laugh silently while making eye contact.
   - Greeting Laughter: Introduce yourselves with hearty laughs instead of words.
   - Lion Laughter: Stick out your tongue, widen your eyes, stretch your hands like claws, and laugh heartily.

4. **Cool Down:**
   - Inhale deeply, hold, and exhale slowly to calm down.
   - Sit quietly for a few minutes, focusing on your breath and relaxation.

5. **Take a moment to thank each other for the session by sharing a big smile with each other.**

Just like the yawning, laughing yoga can activate your mirror neurons. This is what is actually more likely to make you laugh when your partner laughs. This can be a beautiful and positive bonding experience with another person, creating a sense of feeling connected and releasing endorphins.

5. Inner Child Dialogue

When we experience difficult or even traumatic situations as children, we need comfort and support from our caregivers and parents. We need our feelings to be validated, to feel like we are being held, and to know that everything will be okay. If this generally does not happen when we are children, we may start to question or suppress our own feelings, and suffer from helplessness and overwhelm. Over time, as we grow to become adults, we may mask our fears and helplessness by being avoidant, overly confident, and even mean and aggressive. Many people actually don't know how to deal with these more difficult emotions as they arise, so it makes perfect sense why so many people turn to unhealthy coping mechanisms, like substances, overeating or heavy media consumption.

What if there was a way where you could give that younger version of yourself exactly what you would have needed from your parents and caregivers as a child? There is the so-called inner child dialogue. Working with your inner child basically means addressing parts of yourself that have not yet fully emotionally or mentally matured. There are entire books written on this topic, so here I will only quickly mention this practice and how a professional or even a friend can support you.

The main question for having a dialogue with your inner child is to find out what that younger version of you would have needed back in a very specific situation, and provide that to yourself now. The assumption is that we still attempt to somehow fill those needs that were not sufficiently met by your parents or caregivers through others today. This sometimes works, but oftentimes it creates difficulties in interpersonal relations. You can do the following practice by yourself, with a licensed professional or with a compassionate friend you trust.

1. Ensure you feel relatively grounded and emotionally stable when starting this practice. You can begin by imagining a situation of light or medium intensity where you feel your needs were not met by your parents.

2. Ask yourself or have your friend ask you what you would have needed in that specific situation. If you are having difficulties answering this question, think what actions or words would have supported you.

Write these down here.

Words:

_____

_____

_____

_____

Actions:

_____

_____

_____

_____

3. Now see what you would feel comfortable receiving from your partner at this moment. If you do not have a partner, what can you say or do for yourself that would feel nourishing to the need that was not met?

_____

_____

_____

_____

6. Comforting the Inner Child

It may not be so easy to state what exactly your inner child wants to hear. It can be tricky, especially if you are doing such a practice for the first time. Here is a list of common statements for an inner child dialogue that have supported many of my clients in the past in what is called "re-parenting" ourselves. Read through the list of statements and mark the ones that resonate with you most. Write each of these statements on a separate piece of paper and have a friend or therapist read them out to you one after another.

See which one has the strongest impact on you. Work with this particular statement for some time, until there is less of an emotional response. You can also hang the statement up around your house. If you do not have someone to work with, read the statements to yourself in front of a mirror. You will find that only a few of these statements create a strong emotional reaction.

You are loved.	You deserve to be treated with kindness.
You are safe.	You can ask for help.
You are enough	You can forgive yourself.
You are allowed to take care of your needs.	It's okay to make mistakes.
It's okay to play.	You can do this.
It's okay to express your emotions.	You can trust your instincts.
You can take time to rest.	Your feelings matter.
You deserve happiness.	You are allowed to say no.
It's okay to ask questions.	You can walk your own path.
You are resilient.	You have a voice.
You are not alone.	You deserve respect.
It's okay to listen to your body.	You are brave.
You can change your mind.	You have potential.

7. Exploring Different Ways of Co-Regulation Through Touch

Touch is a powerful tool for co-regulation, helping to activate the parasympathetic nervous system and promote feelings of safety and connection. It can help someone out of parasympathetic freeze and out of sympathetic activation. Since touch can be highly triggering for someone that has experienced some form of physical abuse or violence, it should only be used in a careful and consensual manner. If you are supporting someone as a therapist or professional, never touch a client without asking first. Once you begin any practice that involves touch, frequently check in with your client on whether they are still willing to receive your touch. The same goes if you are supporting a friend or partner.

Here are different ways you can use touch to help you or someone else co-regulate. Note that most of the practices involving touch are best done with someone you know personally and trust. Read through the list and then choose to practice the one that feels most appropriate for you at this moment.

1. **Receiving touch from someone we know and trust:**

   - **Sitting Close:** Simply sitting close to someone you trust can provide a sense of safety and connection.

   - **Leaning Against Each Other:** Leaning back-to-back or side-to-side can create a shared sense of calm.

   - **Gentle Hand Holding:** Holding hands with a trusted person can provide immediate comfort and signal safety to your nervous system.

   - **Head Patting:** Gently patting someone's head can be very soothing.

   - **Back Rubbing:** Gentle back rubs can help relax the muscles and signal safety to the nervous system.

   - **Arm Stroking:** Lightly stroking someone's arm can help them feel more relaxed and connected.

   - **Shoulder Massage:** A gentle shoulder massage can release tension and promote relaxation.

   - **Foot Massage:** Foot massages can help ground and calm both the giver and receiver.

   - **Long Hugs:** Engaging in hugs that last at least 20 seconds stimulates the release of oxytocin, which helps reduce stress and enhance feelings of safety and bonding.

   - **Heart-to-Heart Hugs:** Aligning your chest with someone else's can enhance the calming effect of the hug.

   - **Cuddle Sessions:** Spending time cuddling with a partner or loved one can significantly reduce stress and anxiety.

   - **Weighted Blankets:** While not the touch of another person, weighted blankets can simulate the feeling of being held and help calm the nervous system.

2. **Receiving touch from a therapist or licensed professional:**

- Placing hands on the client's shoulder or tapping their back.
- Any form of alternative healing, such as massage, Reiki or energy healing, acupuncture or craniosacral therapy.

8. Combining Touch with Different Cues

I have mentioned throughout this workbook that people with trauma, PTSD or C-PTSD often perceive the world differently. The perception of faces and voices changes, often resulting in seeing and hearing danger where there actually is none. If someone does not learn to co-regulate through their parents or caregivers, is met with inconsistent emotional or physical availability or is even a victim of abuse in their own home, their ability to connect with others is often disturbed. Living in a constant state of dysregulation of the nervous system, whether it's freeze/collapse or fight/flight, will reduce your capacity to feel calm and at ease around others. Yet, it is the relationships with others that can really help bring the nervous system back into a regulated state. Imagine you were bullied at school. You were quite smart and much more interested in books and philosophical discussions with the teacher than being cool and getting along with others. You are left out and are often verbally the target of the "cool" kids in class. Furthermore, you learn that it's not safe to be around others, especially if you are being yourself.

20 years later, you still have problems connecting to others. You don't know how to behave and assume that if you act like yourself you will be rejected. As a result, you continue to spend most of your time alone, making it harder and harder for others to approach you. How do you presume you can heal this teenage trauma? The only way to heal your insecurity and fear of rejection is exactly through social contact with others. Contact people who unconditionally accept you just the way you are,people who help you see that you are loved and accepted no matter what. Here are a few more inspirations to the touch practices.

Practice Facial Cues and Voice Tone with Touch

Go back to the previous tool and pick a way of receiving a form of touch you haven't tried from someone that you love and trust. Practice with a partner, and ask them to include some facial cues. It's best to pick one of the practices where you can actually see each other for this. Ask your partner to smile gently and maintain eye contact while supporting you with their touch.

Ensure that you only do this practice if you feel okay with being touched at this moment. As a therapist, it is best to work with facial cues and voice tone before moving to a practice of co-regulation through touch. You can support your clients through a gentle smile and a soft, calm voice, stating things such as "That must have been difficult for you," or "I can understand your anger."

9. Co-Regulation Through Touch: A Big Strong Hug

Since touch is such an important way to help someone regulate and calm their nervous system, I would like to share another method that can work well between a couple, very good friends or close family members. Ensure that you practice this method at a time when you are calm and relaxed. Then ask your friends to support you the next time they see you emotional or upset.

You can either ask your friend to perform a big strong hug facing you or from behind while either standing up or sitting. Make sure you choose what feels best and most supportive for you. In a moment when you feel upset or emotional, your close friend, family member or partner will begin to hug you in the way you practiced before. They will hug you as hard as you tell them to, but do note that the squeeze is intended to be noticeable. Your partner should hug you for as long as it takes for you to feel quieter and calmer inside.

Note also that there may be some resistance in the beginning, especially if you are experiencing strong emotions. This practice really needs to be done with caution and care, and at the right moment. Also, this practice may not be for everyone. While touch is very supportive for some people in their healing process, too much or unasked for touch can feel absolutely overwhelming for others. As you practice this with someone who is close to you in a calm and relaxed state, really contemplate if this practice is likely to support you in an emotional moment.

10. Co-Regulation Through Breathing Together

Another valuable tool in the series of co-regulation practices is shared breathing with a friend or therapist. This practice involves sitting comfortably facing each other to establish a connection.

- Begin by making gentle eye contact to foster a sense of trust and presence.

- Place one hand on your heart and the other on your friend's or therapist's hand to create a physical link. If you don't feel comfortable touching your therapist, you can also do this practice by simply sitting across from and looking at each other.

- Start breathing slowly and deeply together. Take your time to simply begin synchronizing your breaths.

- Then, after some moments, begin to further synchronize your breath in the following way: Inhale through your nose for a count of four, hold for four, and exhale through your mouth for a count of six.

- Continue this synchronized breathing for a few minutes, focusing on the shared rhythm and the calming presence of each other.

- Gently end the practice after roughly 5 minutes.

- Continue breathing at your own rhythm, while showing each other a little sign of appreciation. End the practice when you both feel ready.

This exercise promotes a deep sense of safety, relaxation and connection, helping you to regulate your nervous system.

11. Re-Storying a Memory

The following practice should be done with extra care, and at a time when you or your client has begun to move into ventral vagal social engagement, or is otherwise feeling grounded and stable. The purpose of this practice is to go through a difficult past experience or memory. It shouldn't be the first time you speak or share about this specific event. Decide for yourself now if you have processed the situation sufficiently, so that speaking about it is not likely to have you feeling helpless, overwhelmed or paralyzed.

The intention of the practice is to reprogram the elements of the incident that you found/find the most difficult. If you are working with a friend or partner, ensure that they can emotionally hold what you are going to share with them. Ideally, you have shared the situation with them in the past. If you have experienced severe trauma, or any forms of sexual or physical abuse, it is best to leave these kinds of practices to be done under the supervision of a therapist or licensed professional. Going back to a traumatic memory or incident without appropriate supervision can make matters worse, causing symptoms to worsen or lead to re-traumatization.

Read the instructions below or listen to the guided audio for this exercise accessible by scanning the following QR code or using this url:
https://bit.ly/ptmadesimple

- Begin the practice by taking some moments to simply breathe deeply together, helping you both become more present with each other. Decide together on certain indicators that are likely to suggest you are overwhelmed and had better stop the practice and switch to a non-verbal form of co-regulation.

- Begin by sharing about the event or situation. Share as much detail as you like and as is needed for you both to fully understand and mentally go to this situation.

- When you get to the difficult moments that have and maybe are still creating difficulties for you in your life, ask your partner to help you support yourself by ensuring that they are there and fully present with you. They can use co-regulation practices, including touch or words of support.

- As you speak of the triggering and traumatic moments, begin to share what you would now say or do to any persons involved. Your partner can encourage you by asking, "What would you like to say to this person?" or "How would you act in this situation today?" If you are having difficulties finding alternative ways of acting, your partner can carefully suggest something.

- Keep sharing about what you would have liked to do or say. You can also include saying things such as "As an adult, I do not tolerate such a behavior," or "This was not ok."

- You can go back into the memory also acting out any behavior with your partner, given of course that you do not hurt yourself or them. If it feels okay for you, you can also choose to create a different ending or outcome of a situation.

- When this practice feels finished and complete, and you feel like you said and did everything, take some deep breaths together. Tell your partner how they can support and comfort you at this time. Ideally, you can go out of this practice feeling a sense of accomplishment and renewed confidence about the event.

- Take a moment to debrief with your partner on anything else about this practice. If there is anything you would have liked or needed to be done differently, share this with your partner.

- Thank each other and show appreciation for the mutual trust, your partners support and your vulnerability.

- Ensure you have quiet, restful time after this practice. Talk together about anything that may arise later as a result of the practice, and journal any insight for a deeper processing.

12. Playful Co-Regulation: Mirror Movements

A playful co-regulation practice for adults with trauma is a practice called "Mirror Movements." This practice helps build trust and connection, and is light-hearted and fun. You will need a partner for this exercise. If you are a therapist or licensed professional, you can practice this with your clients.

1. Sit or stand facing your partner, ensuring you're both comfortable and have enough space.

2. Begin with a few deep breaths together to create a calm atmosphere.

3. Start with the mirror movements: One person starts as the "leader" and the other as the "mirror." The leader makes slow, gentle movements such as raising an arm, tilting their head, or making a silly face. The mirror mimics these actions as closely as possible.

4. After a minute or two, switch roles so you both have the chance to lead and follow.

5. After several rounds, take a moment to discuss how the exercise felt, emphasizing any feelings of connection, safety or joy.

This practice helps build trust and connection while fostering a sense of joy.[29, 30, 31] Remember that healing doesn't always have to be hard and painful. It surely isn't easy, but you are also allowed to have occasional fun. I needed to give many clients of mine permission to also enjoy parts of their healing processes. It's a rollercoaster ride of many ups and downs, not just downs. So a practice that encourages a mutual presence and playful engagement is not only helpful but often needed over the course of an often long healing journey.

13. Playful Co-Regulation: Balloon Breathing

The amount of playful co-regulation partner practices I could list here is endless, really. What's important is that there is an element of interacting together and performing a similar behavior or action. It's helpful when there is a little challenge involved, helping both sides activate parts of the brain that are responsible for logical, reflected action while also engaging areas for motor response and control. Any practices that also activate some form of deeper, more conscious breathing ensure the automatic parasympathetic activation of the nervous system, helping you feel more calm and relaxed.

1. Begin the practice with your partner, facing each other. Take a moment to ground yourself and just arrive in this moment together. You can smile, playfully shake hands or hug each other if you feel comfortable.

2. Then begin to imagine you are both holding a balloon between your hands.

3. Start breathing deeply together by inhaling through your nose and expanding your hands as if inflating the balloon.

4. As you exhale together slowly through your mouth, bring your hands back together as if deflating the balloon.

5. Take turns leading and following, and mirroring each other's breathing and hand movements.

6. You can also pretend the balloon changes colors or shapes over time.

Notice that these playful exercises are also great for practicing co-regulation with children. As simple as this practice sounds, it fosters a sense of togetherness while being mindful and connected. For therapists that are working with clients, the size and shape of the balloon can also symbolize the perceived difficulties or challenges at any moment. So when you sense that your client is really struggling at a certain point, you can use this practice to invite them to actively reform and re-shape their current experience by decreasing the balloon in size.

14. Silent Charades

The way back into ventral vagal social engagement is, for some, very natural. For others, social connections have been more tricky in the past, or someone generally prefers more silence and even solitude. Please note that while this last chapter emphasized the importance of social connections, the chapter does not suggest that you should always be in the presence of others. Everyone has a different preference for spending time with others. Yet, for most, social engagement is a sign of stability and health. If you are one of the quieter ones, you might have fewer friends to meet or engage with. Yet even for those needing less social connections, social engagement is usually crucial to healing.

So, coming to the end of this workbook (one more powerful tool awaits after this one), I invite you to another little playful practice with a partner. This practice works great when working with clients or patients, as it enhances connection through a shared focus and task, and can help improve non-verbal communication and empathy while promoting laughter and fun. Here's how you can do this practice:

1. Prepare a list of words or phrases to act out and prepare a timer. Take about 10–15 minutes for this practice. Start with a few minutes of deep breathing together.

2. One person acts out a word or phrase without speaking, while the other guesses it within a set time limit.

3. Take turns and keep track of how long it takes for you to guess a word or phrase.

4. Reflect on the experience, discussing how it felt to communicate non-verbally and any insights gained.

15. Connection with Gratitude

The last practice of this chapter and workbook can be done in the presence of a dear friend or together with your therapist, and is intended to help you develop a deeper trust and connection, despite any painful or traumatic memories of experiences of the past. There is this saying that we cannot change what happened to us in the past, but we can change how we react to any given circumstance and what we do in the future. Every time we can connect with this sense of confidence and trust that we have this choice, we are likely to feel more optimistic about the future and our paths. This sense of deeper trust and, at times, going beyond all the experiences and memories that shaped us, can help us connect with something greater than ourselves.

For this final practice, I invite you to connect with this sense of deeper connection and gratitude for life, to remember that you are more than just your memories or experiences.

If you like, you can practice together with a dear friend or spouse. Ensure that you are in a space where you feel calm and at peace and can relax while not being disturbed for at least 5 minutes. If you have a candle or even any incense, feel free to light it. Create an atmosphere that evokes lightness and connection. Play some gentle, inspiring music if you like. Read the instructions below or listen to the guided audio for this exercise accessible by scanning the following QR code or using this url: *https://bit.ly/ptmadesimple*

Come to sit or lie down, ensuring you will be comfortable for the next 5 minutes.

- Take a few very deep breaths. With every exhale, release tension, stress and negative thoughts.

- Eventually, place your right hand over your heart while resting your left by your side or on your knees. Deeply breathe into your heart a few times.

- See if you can feel the connection to yourself and evoke a sense of softness in your being. When you feel ready, begin to connect with feelings of gratitude and appreciation for life. See if you can experience any feelings of thankfulness for the people in your life that you love and care for. Evoke feelings of gratitude for yourself and the life you have been given.

- See if you can open your heart just a little bit wider, evoking a sense of gratitude for the earth and expanding your gratitude beyond yourself to something greater than you.

- Rest in these feelings of appreciation, while inviting a sense of trust and confidence in yourself and in your life. If you feel like it, speak out any words of appreciation and thankfulness.

- Slowly finish the practice by evoking this sense of trust and connection for your future. Console yourself in any way by giving yourself a hug, allowing any tears that may arise, and going beyond any thoughts and stories of the mind.

- Simply rest in trust, confidence and gratitude.

- End the practice at your own time and when you feel ready.

Journal any insights and note down the things you appreciate and are grateful for.

_____

_____

_____

_____

Conclusion

The polyvagal theory and the integration of the nervous system responses, and the vagus nerve into therapy are some very promising therapeutic interventions of the past decades. Vagus nerve stimulators have been used for decades and are now proven to effectively support patients with epilepsy and depression.32 Other illnesses, such as PTSD, are under investigation. It is a positive development that speaking about and addressing trauma, PTSD, C-PTSD and many other psychological illnesses has become much more normalized over the past years, as we see the effects of adverse childhood experiences and difficult life events not just in distant third world countries, but all around us.

PVT reminds practitioners and clients of the importance of seeing health on a holistic and integrated level. PVT invites patients and clients back into a relationship with their bodies, helping people understand and experience the innate wisdom of them. As our bodies are wired for survival, whatever we experience in life, our bodies will ensure exactly this. Sometimes this is beneficial and allows us to act quickly in critical moments, such as an accident on the road right in front of us.

While classic therapy targets the mind for healing, somatic therapy and PVT first work with the body, while only later incorporating the mind. PVT allows people to move through and release the stress and charges they have accumulated over the course of their lives, especially those from traumatic memories and events.

In moments of intense distress and activation, our bodies react more than our minds. PVT and integrating the vagus nerve is a practical, somatic approach that can help you heal at the level of body, mind and emotions, harmonizing and regulating the nervous system responses and helping you better navigate the challenges of life.

I truly hope that this workbook and the presented practices, ideas and examples support you on your healing journey, and that you keep this book as a helpful reference and toolbox for the future. May this workbook have inspired and motivated you to move on your personal healing path with confidence, trust and a deeper gratitude. May you be reminded that, despite any setbacks you may encounter throughout life, you should never forget that life is truly a gift.

Before Continuing
Your Journey

Thank you for taking the time to go through this book I sincerely hope the exercises have been beneficial to you.

I have a question, would you be willing to help someone else discover this too if all it cost was less than 60 seconds of your time?

If you would that's amazing! All you have to do is give an honest review on Amazon for this book. It's a simple act but for small publishers it provides an incredible amount of support.

It would be more than worth it if it could help even just one more person struggling with past trauma, anxiety, or depression.

To do that, and to keep it as quick and easy as possible, please click the link below or scan a QR code with your cell phone's camera and press the link that comes up to go directly to your amazon review page.

Another option if you don't want to use the link is to head to your Amazon orders page, locate this book, and and click the "Write a Product Review" option.

Thank you so much for your time. It really does go a long way towards helping more people discover polyvagal theory and these resources.

Endnotes

1   What is Polyvagal Theory | Polyvagal Institute. (n.d.). Polyvagal Institute. *https://www.polyvagalinstitute.org/whatispolyvagaltheory*

2   Porges, S. W. (2022). Polyvagal Theory: A Science of safety. Frontiers in Integrative Neuroscience, 16. *https://doi.org/10.3389/fnint.2022.871227*

3   Smyth, J. M., Johnson, J. A., Auer, B. J., Lehman, E., Talamo, G., & Sciamanna, C. N. (2018). Online Positive Affect Journaling in the Improvement of Mental Distress and Well-Being in General medical patients with Elevated Anxiety Symptoms: a preliminary randomized controlled trial. JMIR Mental Health, 5(4), e11290. *https://doi.org/10.2196/11290*

4   Ashley, V., & Swick, D. (2019). Angry and fearful face conflict effects in post-traumatic stress disorder. Frontiers in Psychology, 10. *https://doi.org/10.3389/fpsyg.2019.00136*

5   Calm Editorial Team. (2024, February 9). How shallow breathing affects the body and mind — Calm Blog. Calm Blog. *https://www.calm.com/blog/shallow-breathing*

6   WebMD Editorial Contributors. (2023, April 30). What is box breathing? WebMD. *https://www.webmd.com/balance/what-is-box-breathing*

7   Ramesh, A., Nayak, T., Beestrum, M., Quer, G., & Pandit, J. (2023). Heart Rate Variability in Psychiatric Disorders: A Systematic review. Neuropsychiatric Disease and Treatment, Volume 19, 2217–2239. *https://doi.org/10.2147/ndt.s429592*

8   Meditation to Boost Health and Well-Being. (2024, January 25). *www.heart.org. https://www.heart.org/en/healthy-living/healthy-lifestyle/mental-health-and-wellbeing/meditation-to-boost-health-and-wellbeing*

9   Sinha, A. N., Deepak, D., & Gusain, V. S. (2013). Assessment of the effects of Pranayama/Alternate nostril breathing on the parasympathetic nervous system in young adults. Journal of Clinical and Diagnostic Research. *https://doi.org/10.7*

10   Breit, S., Kupferberg, A., Rogler, G., & Hasler, G. (2018). Vagus nerve as modulator of the Brain–Gut axis in psychiatric and inflammatory disorders. Frontiers in Psychiatry, 9. *https://doi.org/10.3389/fpsyt.2018.00044*

11   Good Morning America. (2021, May 24). Prince Harry opens up about EMDR therapy in new show l GMA [Video]. YouTube. *https://www.youtube.com/watch?v=QGiqBazdPGw*. Accessed on 25.06.2024.

12   Dreisoerner, A., Junker, N. M., Schlotz, W., Heimrich, J., Bloemeke, S., Ditzen, B., & Van Dick, R. (2021). Self-soothing touch and being hugged reduce cortisol responses to stress: A randomized controlled trial on stress, physical touch, and social identity. Comprehensive Psychoneuroendocrinology, 8, 100091. *https://doi.org/10.1016/j.cpnec.2021.100091*

13   Haynes, A. C., Lywood, A., Crowe, E. M., Fielding, J. L., Rossiter, J. M., & Kent, C. (2022). A calming hug: Design and validation of a tactile aid to ease anxiety. PloS One, 17(3), e0259838. *https://doi.org/10.1371/journal.pone.0259838*

14   Kolk, V. D., & Bessel, A. (2014). The body keeps the score: brain, mind, and body in the healing of trauma. *https://ci.nii.ac.jp/ncid/BB19708339*

15   Kraushaar, S. (2019). Hug Therapy: A 21-Day Journey to Embracing Yourself, Your Life, and Everyone Around You. Mango Media Inc.

16   Lifting weights makes your nervous system stronger too. (2021, March 3). Press Office. *https://www.ncl.ac.uk/press/articles/archive/2020/06/lifting-weightsmakesyournervoussystemstronger/*

17   Zaatar, M. T., Alhakim, K., Enayeh, M., & Tamer, R. (2024). The transformative power of music: Insights into neuroplasticity, health, and disease. Brain, Behavior, & Immunity. Health, 35, 100716. *https://doi.org/10.1016/j.bbih.2023.100716*

18   Ottani, A., Giuliani, D., Galantucci, M., Spaccapelo, L., Novellino, E., Grieco, P., Jochem, J., & Guarini, S. (2010). Melanocortins counteract inflammatory and apoptotic responses to prolonged myocardial ischemia/reperfusion through a vagus nerve-mediated mechanism. European Journal of Pharmacology, 637(1–3), 124–130. *https://doi.org/10.1016/j.ejphar.2010.03.052*

19   Buczynski, R., PhD. (2022). How to help your clients understand their window of tolerance. NICABM. *https://www.nicabm.com/trauma-how-to-help-your-clients-understand-their-window-of-tolerance/*

20   Levine, P. A. (1997). Waking the tiger - healing trauma - the innate capacity to transform overwhelming experiences. In North Atlantic Books. *http://ci.nii.ac.jp/ncid/BA69201502*

21   Huberman, A. (2021). "How to Control Your Stress in Real-Time." Huberman Lab Podcast.

22   Anae. (2016, February 3). Fractals in psychology and art | Richard Taylor. *https://blogs.uoregon.edu/richardtaylor/2016/02/03/human-physiological-responses-to-fractals-in-nature-and-art/*

23   Bradt, J., & Dileo, C. (2014). Music interventions for mechanically ventilated patients. The Cochrane Database of Systematic Reviews, (12), CD006902. doi:10.1002/14651858.CD006902.pub3

24   Benfield, J. A., Taff, B. D., Newman, P., & Smyth, J. (2014). Natural sound facilitates mood recovery. Ecopsychology, 6(3), 183-188. doi:10.1089/eco.2014.0028

25   Harvard Health. (2011, January 18). Strengthen relationships for longer, healthier life. *https://www.health.harvard.edu/healthbeat/strengthen-relation-ships-for-longer-healthier-life*

26   Young, S. N. (2008, September 1). The neurobiology of human social behaviour: an important but neglected topic. PubMed Central (PMC). *https://www.ncbi.nlm.nih.gov/pmc/articles/PMC2527715/*

27   Young, S. N. (2008, September 1). The neurobiology of human social behaviour: an important but neglected topic. PubMed Central (PMC). *https://www.ncbi.nlm.nih.gov/pmc/articles/PMC2527715/*

28   ÇeliK, A. S., & Kılınç, T. (2022). The effect of laughter yoga on perceived stress, burnout, and life satisfaction in nurses during the pandemic: A randomized controlled trial. Complementary Therapies in Clinical Practice, 49, 101637. *https://doi.org/10.1016/j.ctcp.2022.101637*

29   Porges, S. W. (2011). The Polyvagal Theory: Neurophysiological Foundations of Emotions, Attachment, Communication, and Self-Regulation. W.W. Norton & Company.

30   Siegel, D. J. (2012). The Developing Mind: How Relationships and the Brain Interact to Shape Who We Are. The Guilford Press.

31   Brown, S. (2009). Play: How It Shapes the Brain, Opens the Imagination, and Invigorates the Soul. Avery.

32   Abdennadher, M., Rohatgi, P., & Saxena, A. (2024). Vagus Nerve Stimulation therapy in Epilepsy: An Overview of technical and surgical method, patient selection, and treatment outcomes. Brain Sciences, 14(7), 675. *https://doi.org/10.3390/brainsci14070675*

Printed in Great Britain
by Amazon

49932869R00089